Praise for *Love Sex and Every*

"This book for the lay person written by Dr Martha Lee fulfills its intended objective of being truly an idiot's guide book for the person coming to terms with his or her own sexuality and learning to handle all aspects of,normal human sexual responses and disorders throughout one's life.

"Her comfortable easy style and simple jargon-free prose steers the reader through the mysteries of human sexuality and advises them on how to identify the myriad sexual and sexuality problems they face. Although both male and female aspects are covered, being a female herself, she clearly reaches out to the women with sexual problems far more easily than a male can hope to accomplish.

"This author is to be congratulated on this excellent work which will clearly find ready readership as there is no equivalent work for the lay person that so clearly gives all the answers to so many questions that we all want to ask but heitheto were afraid of doing so. The crying need for such a book is over. We owe a deep gratitude indeed to her for this valuable made-in-Singapore educational effort from which the ordinary person will be the ultimate beneficiary."

Professor Peter Lim Huat Chye, MD
Senior Consultant & Urological Surgeon
Founder, Society for Men's Health Singapore
Founder, Asian Society for Female Urology

"In her book, Dr Martha Lee has exhibited her deep and profound understanding of the multi-faceted topic that is sexual health by providing clear and easily understandable explanations to what must appear to others as enigmas. The questions in her FAQ format will certainly resonate with many who are seeking clarity on their own sexuality and sexual health and to understand the sexual needs of their partners. This book is thoroughly engaging and readable with anecdotes from Dr Lee's personal experiences and also that of her multitude of patients. I definitely would recommend this book to anyone seeking a deeper insight into human sexuality."

Dr Tan Kok Kuan
Chief Medical Officer
Dr Tan & Partners

"Dr Martha Lee's dedication and sense of purpose that drives her to fulfill her life's work is truly inspiring. Martha's integrity and passion shines through in everything she does and her book is no exception. Her intelligent, candid and compassionate pragmatism makes even this sensitive subject accessible to everyone. I have met very few people with Martha's gift for bringing both scientific rationale and a depth of understanding of the very roots of humanity together. Dr Martha's insights are heartfelt and practical—this book is a must-read for anyone seeking better understanding of intimacy and sexuality."

Gina Romero
Managing Director
The Athena Network Singapore & APAC

"I have been following the work of Dr Martha Tara Lee since she became the first qualified sexologist in Singapore. I am so proud and impressed with her numerous achievements to date—and now her much anticipated first book! Martha is honest, humorous and humble through it all and truly a rising star in the field of sexology. Her personality shines through in this book as does her comprehensive knowledge about sexual health and pleasure. You will find this an enjoyable and educational read—from her insights relating to sex and sexuality, frequently asked questions, to her personal stories."

Dr Patti Britton
Pioneering Sex Coach & Clinical Sexologist
Co-Founder of SexCoachU.com
Author of The Art of Sex Coaching

LOVE
SEX and
EVERYTHING
IN-BETWEEN

Fact and Fiction
from a Sexologist

DR MARTHA TARA LEE

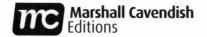

Marshall Cavendish
Editions

Cover design by Benson Tan

© Marshall Cavendish International (Asia) Pte Ltd
Published in 2014 by Marshall Cavendish Editions
An imprint of Marshall Cavendish International
1 New Industrial Road, Singapore 536196

Other Marshall Cavendish Offices:
Marshall Cavendish Corporation. 99 White Plains Road, Tarrytown NY 10591-9001, USA • Marshall Cavendish International (Thailand) Co Ltd. 253 Asoke, 12th Flr, Sukhumvit 21 Road, Klongtoey Nua, Wattana, Bangkok 10110, Thailand • Marshall Cavendish (Malaysia) Sdn Bhd, Times Subang, Lot 46, Subang Hi-Tech Industrial Park, Batu Tiga, 40000 Shah Alam, Selangor Darul Ehsan, Malaysia.

Marshall Cavendish is a trademark of Times Publishing Limited

National Library Board, Singapore Cataloguing-in-Publication Data
Lee, Martha Tara.
Love, sex and everything in-between / Dr Martha Tara Lee.—Singapore : Marshall Cavendish Editions, 2013.
pages cm
ISBN : 978-981-4484-19-0 (paperback)
1. Sex customs. 2. Sexology. 3. Sex instruction. 4. Love.

HQ31
613.9071—dc23   OCN 857866314

Printed in Singapore by Markono Print Media Pte Ltd

Contents

Why I Became a Sexologist

I do this work because there is nothing else I rather be doing. Four years ago, I remember a fellow sexologist asking on an online forum if we should encourage people to pursue sexology as a career.

I responded: "The work that we do is incredibly difficult and often thankless. To me, it is a calling and I do it because I cannot see myself doing anything else. I cannot speak for other people."

Prior to being a sexologist, I worked in corporate communications for eight years—doing public relations, marketing and advertising. I left a comfortable career to do non-profit work, helping young people in the area of career guidance. I was no longer satisfied with the status quo. I could no longer deny that I cared more about people than money, and helping people was more important to me than climbing the corporate ladder. I broke out of my comfort zone and there was no turning back. And yes, it was scary.

After two years of doing volunteer recruitment and management, fundraising and everything in between, I realised my heart was with working with people directly. To "help" from a distance was safe for me and I knew it. I had to put myself on the line.

I had been a volunteer counsellor for three years by then, and realised that there was a jarring gap in the dialogues revolving around sexuality in Singapore.

Before becoming a sexologist, I questioned why nobody was acknowledging the importance of sex and sexuality to one's sense of well-being, not to mention the role it plays in a relationship. Surely, there was more to understanding sex and sexuality than learning to protect against sexually transmitted infections (STIs), making babies and getting your period?

I recognised that there was a lack of any real and meaningful conversations about sex and sexuality. If sex was this wonderful, beautiful and intimate act between two people in love, why is it always talked about so negatively?

The attitude Singaporeans have towards sex have a lot to do with the societal and media messages we are inundated with, not to mention influenced by our culture, religion and parents. Singaporeans seem to be anxious about what is "normal", "correct" and "acceptable"—from length and size of anatomical parts, to sexual frequency, duration and positioning. If there were more accurate and positive sexual information and education available, many sexual concerns would not take on a life of its own or seem bigger than they actually are.

Being a sexologist allows me to be communicator, advocate, coach, teacher and healer all in one. It is a sum of everything I have studied in school, learned in life, and experienced as a human, woman, daughter and wife. My work is pure heart work, and is also hard work(!). It is the product of my desire to leave a legacy of people who are fearlessly living and embracing life fully behind.

I would like to see Singaporeans acknowledging and accepting that our sexuality forms an important part of our sense of being, and begin to dialogue openly, honestly and without guilt or shame. Singaporeans can and ought to take ownership of their sexual pleasure, the same way they tackle the different areas of their life such as family and work. All are important. When they can recognise this, they will naturally take personal responsibility and decisive actions.

Therefore, I am hard-pressed to encourage or persuade anyone to be a sexologist. I am me, and you are you. Our journeys might well be different or similar. Either way, it is all good. It is more important that you find what makes your soul sing, as being a sexologist does for me.

Sex is not everything. But sex is important.

I became a Clinical Sexologist because I had to.

What a Sexologist is Not

I am a sexologist. Since I am the only one at this time with this unique combination of qualification and training in Singapore, there exists a lot of confusion about what exactly a sexologist *does* within our little city-state. Not only that, I have my share of detractors who think I am a "joke", only about hype, or out to create trouble or controversy for the purpose of my own aggrandisement, etc.

I have never professed to be something I am not. Since I am 100% serious about the work I do and intend to be around for some time, here are a few common misconceptions I would like to address:

1. **I do not have a PhD**

   A lot of people think any degree that starts with the word "Doctorate" is a PhD. My school, the Institute for Advanced Study of Human Sexuality, offers five different graduate degrees, including a PhD programme. I chose not to complete a PhD because I did not and probably never will pursue an academic or research-based career. What I have is a Doctorate in Human Sexuality.

2. **I am not a sex therapist**

   While I have a certificate in sex therapy from Florida Sex Therapy Institute, I am not qualified to call myself a sex therapist. A sex therapist, at least in the United States, is somebody who has a psychology degree with a specialisation in sex therapy. In short, a sex therapist is a psychologist first, who subsequently obtains additional training in sex therapy. The training of a sex therapist and one who has studied human sexuality is different. The former looks at sexual difficulties from only the psychological (mind-based) perspective, while a sexologist addresses issues from a more holistic view (i.e. the roles and impact of the body-mind-heart-spirit).

The field of sexology is not one singular discipline, but actually draws upon many disciplines, such as sociology, psychology, anthropology, medicine, and the arts of understanding the various manifestations of human sexuality.

3. I am not a psychologist

Few psychologists or psychotherapists ever get specialised training in human sexuality. The governing body for psychologists in Singapore is the Singapore Psychological Association.

4. I am not a counsellor

You may be able to cook, but it doesn't necessarily make you a chef. Even though I have a certificate in counselling, I do not call myself a counsellor. However, I do use counselling techniques in my practice. The

governing body for counsellors in Singapore is the
Singapore Association for Counselling.

5. **I am not a social worker**

   According the website of the governing body of social
   workers, Singapore Association of Social Workers, social
   workers are primarily dedicated to: assisting people to
   manage their problems more effectively; improving
   social conditions; advocating for change when change is
   necessary to better human lives. I only focus on sexuality
   and intimacy issues and the concerns of individuals and
   couples about these matters.

6. **I am not a medical doctor**

   I do not issue prescriptions, give medication or prescribe
   any kind of drugs. I also do not carry out any physical
   examinations. I do possess some knowledge about the
   kinds of medical drugs that can help sexual difficulties,
   as well as know a whole lot about the types of condoms,
   lubrication, as well as sex toys that people can use. It
   might be worthwhile noting that not all medical doctors
   are trained about the myriad of different sexuality issues
   that people have, and therefore are not familiar with
   them and with talking with their patients about same.

7. **I am not a Tantrica**

   Most Tantra teachers and workshops teach a small
   segment of the Tantric philosophy that focuses on

sexuality, massage and breathing. While I incorporate some Tantric ideas and methods into my work, I neither believe that any kind of sexual expression is the best or only method, nor insist that you adopt a new language or complicated types of breathing. I am not against Tantra. I am just not qualified to teach Tantra.

8. I do not call myself a sexuality educator

I carry out sexuality education all the time—by way of the articles I write for the media, the posts on my blog, Facebook, Twitter, not to mention through my workshops and client sessions. Since a lot of my time is spent being involved in some aspects of sexual education, why didn't I just call myself a sexuality educator? My client sessions are not always and only about sexuality education, some of it involves helping them to work through a very specific sexual problem. A more accurate term for the myriad of things I do is actually sexologist. I did not pluck the term sexologist out of thin air. It is a legitimate professional title that is more commonly used in the United States.

9. I am not your mother

Go ahead, laugh. Sometimes I feel the need to point out the obvious. I am not going to nag or pester you to do your home assignments so that you can overcome your sexual difficulties and go on to have a more fulfilling life. That's your responsibility. My role is to facilitate and support your growth in the best possible ways, not take over for you.

10. **What I am**

I am a specialist in the area of sexual questions or concerns. I am a certified sexuality educator by AASECT (American Association of Sexuality Educators, Counselors and Therapists) as well as a board-certified sexologist by the American College of Sexologists. I am also a certified hypnotherapist, as well as life coach. I employ a combination of counselling, coaching and sex therapy methods and techniques, sometimes including them all, depending on the concern(s) the client(s) come in with.

I certainly do not proclaim to be all things to everyone. By now, you can appreciate the difference in the type of discipline as well as in the practitioner who is most qualified to help you through your own particular issue. The training of one who calls himself or herself a sex therapist, sex doctor or sexologist can vary greatly. One type of degree or work experience doesn't guarantee that a practitioner will work for you. What is important is for you to understand what their qualifications are, and that he or she offers this information directly and completely.

SEX 101:
It's All in Your
Attitude

Defining Sex, Sexuality and Intimacy

What are sex, sexuality and intimacy to you? What do those words actually signify in your mind? Is sex just about the physical act of sexual intercourse? The meaning of "sex" can be problematic when the way you define it is different from the way other people around you do. Not only that, these problems with definition may inadvertently lead to problems with sex. Therefore, it may be useful to take some time to clarify, so that we know what we are talking about when we talk about sex.

What is sex?

Sex is sometimes approached from the biological perspective: a way of distinguishing male and female members of a species. Or, it might simply refer to the genitals. The third definition, the more common one: sexual intercourse, otherwise known as coitus, an act that can result in reproduction between a heterosexual pair.

Having understood the dictionary definition, I would like to contribute my own. Sexual activity, to me, is not only about penile-vaginal penetration. Sex is a result of any sexual stimulation resulting in physiological changes in one or more persons. Hence, hand jobs, blow jobs, foreplay, afterplay, anal touch, porn watching, solo sex or masturbation are all sex to me. Massage may also be sex depending on the way it is delivered, and how it feels for the receiver. Orgasm or ejaculation does not need to take place for sex to have occurred.

Therefore, I would disagree with former United States President Bill Clinton, who, on 26 January 1998, spoke at a White House press conference, and issued a forceful denial, which contained what would later become one of the best-known sound bites of his presidency: "But I want to say one thing to the American people. I want you to listen to me. I'm going to say this again: I did not have sexual relations with that woman, Miss Lewinsky. I never told anybody to lie, not a single time; never. These allegations are false." Clinton later admitted to an improper relationship with Lewinsky, and used a limited, legalistic formulation of the meaning of sex to deny that he lied at this press conference.

To me, sex involves one's entire being—body, mind and emotions. How we think and feel about our bodies, ourselves, and our partners, as well as how we interpret the physical contact, are all dynamics that play out subconsciously during sex. Sex may also be seen as a spiritual act by some—where we are in union with another person.

What is sexuality?

The word sex and sexuality are often used interchangeably. Anna Freud once said, "Sex is something you do, sexuality is something you are."

Sexuality is comprised of more than a sum of the spectrum of sexual activities possible; it is, rather, one's individual sexual expression. As a complex aspect of our personality, it is defined by our sexual thoughts, desires, longings, erotic fantasies, turn-ons, and experiences. Scarleteen, a popular sexuality-resource site, has stated that a person's sexuality is regarded as an intrinsic part of who we are—an identity that cannot be separated any more than our ethnicity, or religious/spiritual beliefs.

Our shame, guilt and/or trauma surrounding sex, our lack of sexuality education, role models and resources about sexuality, as well as our cultural, social and gender expectations all contribute towards this complex picture of what our sexuality becomes. The sexist code embedded in our cultural norms, and sexual stereotypes also play a part in our idea of normal gender roles.

What is intimacy?

Intimacy does not just happen in the bedroom. It is generally agreed that intimacy has to do with the feelings of closeness, safety, and being loved. Intimate behaviours may include being able to share personal feelings, stories, or private thoughts. Being physically close can attribute to greater intimacy, as well as the idea of two people becoming one, or the blurring of subjective boundaries between two different people.

To me, a visual representation of intimacy as seen in my mind's eye involves being able to look across a room full of strangers, catching the gaze of somebody you know at the other end, and being able to instinctively recognise what the other is trying to communicate, whether it's boredom, frustration, or joy. What mental image of intimacy comes up for you?

As you can tell, intimacy is a subjective internal experience requiring at least two individuals. Some people crave more in the way of sexual intimacy than others. A good place to start is to explore for yourself what kinds of sexual intimacy you have experienced in your life thus far, and what you would like more of in the future.

I hope these definitions of sex, sexuality, and intimacy have been useful to you. Share this piece, and discuss the topic with your loved ones. You may be surprised about the difference in views that you encounter.

Dispelling Certain Sexual Myths

Size matters

This has to be the most well-known myth, especially since guys tease or insult each other about being small in size. The penis is a symbol of male identity, sexuality and masculinity, which is why size is often fussed over among men. The notion that a larger penis equates to someone who is more masculine has, in turn, led men to think or feel that bigger is better.

The penises of Singaporean men average 3.5 to 5.9 inches in length. Most men fall somewhere in-between. Size has little to no relation to sexual performance. If he asks you what you think of his penis, know that he is actually asking for reassurance. Encourage him to appreciate his body for what it is—healthy, functioning and perfectly normal.

Men think of sex more often than women

Women want sex as much as men—but they are guided by other emotions as well. A combination of pressures and exhaustion from work and taking care of the household are good enough reasons to go off sex completely.

Hormonal changes and mood swings also make them feel desirable on some days more than others, so they are likely to have a higher sex drive during certain points of the month, rather than crave for sex perpetually.

And like it or not, most women like men to initiate. They are unlikely to beg for sex.

You don't get pregnant while having your period

There is a chance that you can get pregnant during a period, especially towards the tail-end of your menstrual cycle. There are a couple of reasons for this. While having a period means the breaking down of the lining and "washing away", it is possible that an unfertilised egg is still in the uterus and conception can occur if you have sex when you think you are finishing your period.

Ovulation, the process in which a woman's ovaries release an egg, takes place 14 days before the end of your cycle. But when you experience a very short cycle, it is possible that you will ovulate while you are still menstruating. If you have sex before or during your period, then there can be a chance of pregnancy.

Sometimes women who are ovulating can experience vaginal spotting due to stress or hormonal changes, and that can be mistaken for a period. As you are most fertile just after ovulation, you are more likely to get pregnant at this time than any other in your cycle.

Typically, sperm survives for two to three days in a woman's body. But under "optimum" conditions, sperm can stay "active" for up to five days and still be able to fertilise an egg during this time. So if you've had unprotected sex before or after ovulation, it's best you run a pregnancy test.

STI tests are for people cheating on their spouses

Not all sexually transmitted infections (STIs) are sexually transmissible; a number are spread by skin-to-skin contact. For instance, oral herpes may be passed by casual affection between family members. A substantial fraction of people with cold sores get them from their relatives during childhood, but those cold sores can then be spread sexually during oral sex. In addition, many people with STIs have no idea that they are infected, and symptoms may sometimes appear after a couple has been together for years.

Only men enjoy watching porn

According to *The Times of India*, women love porn. UK tabloid, *The Sun*, also reported in 2009 that 66% of women surveyed watch porn.

X-rated films give women new ideas and tricks to experiment with to make their partners happy. Online magazine, Oprah.com stated in an article: "With porn, women get to experiment with making adult choices and trying on new fantasy ideas, just as we might try a different brand of condom for a change."

But *The Sun* reported that women in relationships disliked porn when they catch their partners watching explicit programmes.

Both women and men can use porn to find out what they like and what they are comfortable with in the bedroom.

You can't get pregnant through anal intercourse

It is possible that it could happen if semen from the anus gets into the vagina. With anal sex, STIs are a much bigger worry than pregnancy. The risk of getting an STI like HIV (Human Immunodeficiency Virus) that causes AIDS (Acquired Immunodeficiency Syndrome) is even higher with anal sex than vaginal sex. That's because the lining of the rectum is thin and can tear easily, allowing infection to get into your body.

Two condoms are more effective than one

This act, also known as "double bagging", may seem like a good idea but is NOT! It can actually increase the friction between the condoms during sex which makes them more likely to rip or tear. When used properly, condoms are up to 98% effective and are not only reliable in preventing pregnancy, but can successfully protect against many sexually transmitted infections.

Certain foods such as oysters get you frisky

One thing that brings credibility to the oyster myth is the fact that these are rich in zinc. Zinc controls progesterone levels, which have a positive effect on the libido. Zinc deficiency can cause impotence in men, so any food rich in zinc is considered an aphrodisiac in that respect, and oysters happen to be loaded with the mineral. Because oysters somewhat resemble the female sex organ, this could be a reason why people in the past associated them with sexuality.

The Importance of Listening to Your Emotions

If you accidentally touched a hot stove, the nerves in your skin would send a message of pain to your brain. The brain then sends a message back telling the muscles in your hand to pull away. Is that a bad thing?

No, you would answer. What a ridiculous question, you might retort. Hear me out.

Physical stimuli we receive, or thoughts we have, produce physiological responses as well as further thoughts which tell us how to react to a situation. By adulthood we learn to become pretty good at discerning what is good or bad for us physically. We listen to the safety messages our body sends us.

Yet why do we not listen to what our heart tells us? How can so many people persistently dismiss, deny, or worse, lose touch with their emotions? Our emotions are the result of our mind's interpretation between our bodies and its perceptions of the outside world. Much like the way our physical feelings preserve and ensure our survival, our emotional feelings are developed, refined and perfected through time.

The word "emotion" does not refer to the same thing as "emotional". Yet emotions are usually perceived as a bad thing. We may downplay emotions, seeing it as a sign of weakness. We may even underestimate problems by overlooking negative emotions. Not only that, in denying our feelings and rationalising our problems with our mind, we miss out on real solutions and holistic healing. We are so quick in running away from "bad" feelings that we stand to also lose the renewal that positive emotions can encourage. We are numb. We have lost our true innate ability to survive. Our energy and reserves have run out.

Feelings need not be judged or labelled "good" or "bad". They just are. Negative feelings can warn and help us in particular situations. These are quite normal and necessary for mature behaviour. The inability to express and channel negative feelings is limiting and blocks whole and mature functioning. At its worst, it is crippling. Feelings are often more honest than our minds in telling us "where we are at". It is not an intellectual reply. It is a response that comes from your core—from your gut.

This is why one of the first things a counsellor will do with a new client is to assess how the person feels. Very often, the client themselves is confused about his or her feelings. It is easy enough to verbalise what one thinks consciously, but harder to communicate what one feels from deep within. If there is no congruence between how one feels (emotions), the way one thinks (rational intent), and what one does (volition), a person cannot be whole. An effective counsellor helps to bring these feelings out and facilitates the integration of such feelings into the client's conscious assessment of what is wrong and how one should proceed.

It is helpful to become more aware of your emotional needs as a first step towards self-love. When we become better at identifying and expressing our emotional feelings, we invariably become more socially adept in establishing and building relationships. The more adept we are at identifying and expressing emotional feelings, the better we feel and the better our relationships will be.

I end with a quote by Robert Hendi: "Cherish your emotions and never undervalue them".

Opening Your Heart

To truly "open your heart" to your partner, more than sex is involved. Are you able to be open—which entails being utterly and completely transparent and vulnerable—with your partner? If not, what is preventing you from doing so? Is it the fear of abandonment or rejection? How about the fear of losing oneself? What exactly is it about getting close to someone that is so scary?

Understanding intimacy?

If you look at the word "intimacy" phonetically, you could break it down into "In-To-Me-See". Indeed it is about removing your protective layers and facades, revealing yourself, connecting mentally, emotionally and sexually with your partner, perhaps getting to know each other all over again, exploring non-sexual areas, before working up to primary erogenous zones such as breasts and genitals.

It is about being connected, even from across a room of strangers. Sex without intimacy eventually becomes shallow and unfulfilling. If intimacy is not nurtured, the relationship will wither and die over time.

The deeper your intimacy is in your relationship, the more satisfying the sex will be. When sex is explosive and mind-blowing, it cements you to your lover in a very powerful way, and thus opens the door for more intimacy. Thus, intimacy and great sex feed each other.

Why is there a need for greater intimacy?

A lot of relationships fall apart or the sex within them is not very good anymore because couples have fallen into a rut and begin to take each other for granted. Also any kind of abuse—whether physical, emotional, physiological—does affect intimacy. Once the intellectual and emotional sharing in the relationship stops, intimacy and passion in sex will end soon after.

Women need to feel loved, valued, special, intimate and listened to by their partner for sex to be at its best. If she feels these things, she will desire her lover more deeply and be more willing to pleasure her lover in the way he desires. Men also need intimacy, but may not be as aware of this need and it may not be as evident to them in the context of sex.

How does one overcome fear of intimacy?

Heightening your self-awareness and being conscious in releasing your fear is one way.

Try this simple, but effective, approach:

- Sit in a quiet spot, quiet your thoughts and connect within.
- Allow any feelings you have pushed down for a long time to surface.
- Focus on whatever feelings might come up and allow yourself to fully feel them.
- While feelings of anger, pain, fear, shame or sadness might be quite intense, such feelings can dissolve and disappear once you acknowledge them.

The other way is to just take small steps to becoming more intimate. Allow yourself to feel vulnerable enough to talk to your loved one about what is going on in your life and how you really feel about it. Be 100% present and enjoy the process. Indeed, the more you practise self-disclosure, the easier it becomes.

How does one cultivate greater intimacy?

Intimacy has to do with your daily communication—from the way you address each other, how you apologise when at fault, how open you are with most of your daily dealings to the kind of friends that you keep. The first thing is to acknowledge this as a couple, and be conscious of the words you are using and what they mean.

Sharing makes you vulnerable and can feel extremely risky and scary. Most people don't like that and intentionally avoid being vulnerable—perhaps by keeping themselves busy with their career—and thereby run away from intimacy. Also, because you value and cherish the opinion of your spouse, or know your spouse so well that you can anticipate what he or she might say, you refrain from sharing for fear of the reaction and judgement.

When a woman experiences intimacy with her partner, she feels safe and she will surrender herself deeply so she can feel ultimate pleasure and satisfaction without any inhibitions. For a man, intimacy can be better than sex because it takes the pressure off performance and it makes him feel valued by his partner. It takes being open to the experience.

By building intimacy, expressing affection and love, you can begin rediscovering each other and your needs and desires more deeply. You can recapture the same passion and excitement that you felt earlier in your relationship.

Love is precious. We all need to feel love and to feel loved. Don't be afraid of it. Open up your heart and allow love in. It is beautiful.

Greater Intimacy at a Glance

- Build trust and create a safe space to do so. Share your fears. Share your dreams.
- Encourage the other person to do the same.
- Acknowledge each other's fears—having fears validated is profound.
- Keep your eyes open for signs of abuse, imbalance and fear.
- Be ready to back off a little if necessary.

The Importance of Touch

Touch is the medium through which we first become acquainted with the world. It is the first means of communication between a newborn baby and the mother. Research has shown that many babies who are raised in an orphanage and are not handled and touched on a regular basis rarely live past the age of two—they literally wither away.

Some people like to touch others, and some do not. Some like being touched, yet others might not. Are you a toucher or non-toucher? Do you realise that the way your parents held you as a newborn—from the pressures, caresses, to cuddles—influence the way you have developed? And the touch you received as a child through play, punishment and bathing directly relates to your responsiveness as an adult?

Your body remembers. If you were touched often and lovingly as a child, you are much more likely to be comfortable experiencing the pleasure of your lover's touch. If, however, your memories of being touched bring forth memories of punishment, rejection or pain, your body will inadvertently withdraw from touch, fearing further hurt. This is where you might like to seek out therapeutic approaches such as counselling or massage for physical memory healing.

It's not uncommon for one partner to need more physical connection than the other. Studies have shown that touch can lower stress levels, lessen anxiety, and help a myriad of other physical disorders. There are noticeable changes in mood and even health when we're exposed to simple human kindness in the form of touch.

If you yearn for physical closeness, be it a hug or a snuggle, communicate your need to your partner. If a hug is all you want, clearly communicate this. The desire for physical closeness often gets misinterpreted as a desire for sex. Misunderstandings that stem from miscommunication about how we want, like or need to be touched does happen. So, communicate, communicate and communicate!

Also, if you desire more touch in your relationship, acknowledge that you feel less connected and want a way to spend more time touching him or her, and helping the other person feel loved.

Physical closeness and touching stimulates the continued growth of your loving relationships. It is the conduit between two individuals that allows them to connect as one. You can:

- Hug and kiss each other before you leave for work, or when you return home.
- Give affection to each other during quiet moments of the day.
- Hold hands while walking down the street, watching a movie or between courses at a restaurant.
- Shower or bathe together. (It helps the two of you feel emotionally closer, and also become physically cleaner!)
- Ask for a massage and give one in return.
- Subtly keep your hand on your partner's leg, or on the small of the back, to maintain a physical connection.

Touch establishes communication, and what is transmitted has more meaning than words. Touch communicates involvement. It means you care that you are really supporting the other person. Touch heals and provides emotional sustenance. So reach out and touch your partner today.

Touch Your Partner

The skin: Our skin is our biggest sexual organ. Massage your partner all over—not too hard but firm enough to encourage blood circulation. Vary your touch—from hard pressure on the shoulders with the soft pads of your fingers to light scratching with your nails over their back.

The lips: Build up the sexual tension between the two of you by giving different kinds of kisses. Start off by tracing your index finger over the lips. Ask your partner not to move as you place your lips over his or hers. Don't be afraid to use your tongue to trace the lips and tease your way into his or her mouth. See if the other person doesn't start responding!

The hair: Run your fingers through his or her hair lightly to stimulate what a scalp massage in the shower might feel like. This can be erotic as it helps relax and arouse at the same thing. You may wish to pull his or her hair back slightly as the excitement builds—pain and pressure can go hand in hand.

The ear: Explore around and behind the ears with your tongue softly. Enact what you would do if kissing the lips. You may wish to also suck or pull on the edge of the ears with your lips. Nibble at the ear lobes, breath into the ear and tell your partner how you want him or her.

The neck: The neck and collarbone have lots of nerve endings. Biting and kissing roughly may lead to broken blood vessels and consequently love bites. Run your fingers smoothly along the edges of his collarbone. Licking along the edges of the neck can remind your partner of what is to follow as you head south.

Types of hugs

- A hug that's followed by a thump on the back above or below shoulders is more of a friendly or "hey how have you been" hug. This is an indication of discomfort with hugging you or with your closeness. However not all back thumping is negative and it can be difficult to analyse the precise reason.
- A crushing bear hug can be a more intense variation of a hug. This hug can be the other person's way of outwardly demonstrating the amount of love he or she has for

you. Unless you dislike or object to this type of hug periodically, I'd say enjoy! It sure beats receiving a floppy, half-hearted attempt of a hug, isn't it?

• A hug from behind is romantically inspired. Where one person from behind wraps their arms around the other, it carries sexual connotations and can be intimate.

All in all, regardless of the type of hug you give or receive, a hug is a hug and it carries emotional benefits. Hugs can be heartwarming, therapeutic and give the effect of leaving one energised and rejuvenated

Q *Is there a way to tell when a guy is hugging you as a friend or as someone who's attracted to you? Are there any subtle differences we can pick up on?*

A You might think that a hug is a hug is a hug, but not all hugs are the same. You can tell subtly and perhaps even intuitively or subconsciously that a guy hugging you is doing so as a friend, hoping for more, or romantically attracted to you—from the strength or tenderness of the hug, tension of his body, reluctance to let go, lingering touch, and roaming of the hands below your shoulders. Let's not forget other cues such as eye contact, breathing rate, and heartbeat. But most of all, listen to your gut, your feelings and what your heart says. If you are not comfortable with being hugged or touched by him, ask yourself why. Does it have anything to do with you not liking him romantically?

The Elephant in the Bedroom: Talking about Sex

For most people, sex is a sensitive and difficult subject to talk about.

I have come across a man who, after 15 years of marriage, admitted that he and his wife have never talked about sex. Don't get me wrong. They <u>DO</u> have sex. They just don't talk about it.

In other words, they never talked about their preferences when it comes to sexual position or techniques. And because sex has become the elephant in the bedroom, I would suppose they also have never shared how they would prefer to be touched—much less ask for it. Not only have they not ventured into asking each other for feedback, they would most certainly not be coming up with new ideas of what they would like to do but have not tried any time soon.

One of my favourite sayings goes like this: "If you don't ask for what you want, you will most certainly not get it." But the first thing is to know what it is you want. And how will you know what it is you want or like if you have never tried it?

If sex is as simple as: trying something (be it a position, technique or otherwise); seeing if you like it; doing more of it; being sure of what you want; and then asking for it, why aren't more people doing A, B or C to get D? What is it about S-E-X that is so scary? What is it about our sexuality that we are trying to (or not to) express?

The truth of the matter is: how many of us were exposed to sexuality education growing up? And I don't mean how the sperm meets the egg. I am also not just talking about how women bleed once a month (and the men going 'eek!'), safer sex or STIs. I am referring to honest conversations about all aspects of one's sexuality including: body image, sexual orientation, values, decision-making, communication, dating, relationships, etc. as well as sex as a pleasurable act.

If we haven't had such exposure, just how do we begin to know what it is we don't know, but should know? And just how, with this lack of sexuality education, do we talk about sex in an adult and mature manner? We can't. We want to but do not know how.

At networking events, I have been the butt of many jokes about the nature of my work. Somebody, with X number of kids, will invariably say something to this effect: "Oh I won't be needing any help from you. I have X kids to prove that I have no problems."

Surely sex is more than just reproduction. And just what does it say about one when a person is so quick to dismiss any kind of a conversation related to sexuality?

This brings me back to: For most people, sex is a sensitive and difficult subject to talk about.

Sex is Learned

Sex is a learned act. That's right: l-e-a-r-n-e-d.

I remember contributing an article to an online portal three years ago. I had written the sentence: "For most people, sex is a learned act." When the portal owner's edits come back, she had written: "Don't you mean, 'For most people, sex is a natural act'?".

My immediate response was territorial: "Who is the sexologist here? Are you saying I am wrong? What are you trying to imply here?"

When I calmed down sufficiently, I had to acknowledge that the portal owner wrote what she did because she truly thought she was right. She suspected that I had made a genuine mistake and was only trying to be helpful. I decided to store this story at the back of my head until a more opportune time to share my views arrived.

If sex was supposed to be natural, easy and effortless between two persons in love, how would it explain the couples who seek my support, unsure of how to consummate their marriage? Are they any less in love?

If sex was natural, why do people still have fears, anxieties, concerns and questions about sex?

If sex was natural, why are there people who do not like, do not want, or do not desire sex?

Are these people (gasp!) unnatural beings?

Case in point, one of the most comfortable sexual positions for a woman is when she lifts both her legs in the air and spreads her legs wide apart as her partner mounts her. This is known as the missionary position. For the longest time, I felt like, and I swear looked like, a frog. If sex is supposed to be natural, it most certainly didn't feel like it. And it didn't become "natural" for a while.

Didn't it occur to the above-mentioned portal owner that what she feels is natural sexually is also learned?

The first people we learn about sexuality from are our parents, from the answer to our question "Where did I come from?" As we enter school, our sexual information might increasingly come from our classmates. When we reach adolescence, other sources of information may include the media such as the Internet, movies, books and maybe whatever online porn you could get a hold of (even though you are not supposed to). If you were lucky, you might have received some sexual education in school—never mind the quality or depth of it.

Like much of everything we know, we acquire the knowledge, practiSe through trial and error, and perfect it so that it becomes a skill which we "own". Hence, the word: "sexual skill". Sex is a skill. Sex involves sexual techniques.

One can certainly buy sexual educational books in shrink-wrapped plastic from the bookshops. Or attend one of my many sexual technique workshops.

Yes, my friend, sex is not a natural act. It is learned.

Sex is Not the Same as Studying from the 10-year-series

I tell my clients that sex is not the same as studying from the 10-year-series. For those who don't know, the 10-year-series is a colloquial term unique to Singapore, where students refer to official compilations of examination papers from past years for the GCE N-levels, O-levels and A-levels, approved by the Ministry of Education and University of Cambridge Local Examination Syndicate, respectively.

One should not compare sex with sitting for a school examination, but I am just about to.

For exam questions, there is a model answer. We are talking about absolutes—you are either right or wrong. There is a set of perfect answers and the goal is to get a hundred out of a hundred. You could do very well, well, pass or fail.

And you have guessed what I am going to say: sex is not about that.

There are no absolutes when it comes to sex. There is no right or wrong. There is rarely, if ever, a perfect lovemaking session. Sure you can have a great, fantastic, even mind-blowing lovemaking session, but it might never be perfect.

Why? Because we are all unique individuals who have different bodies, sexual responses, and preferences, which (gasp!) might change on a day-to-day basis depending on many factors. These might include our stress, tiredness or fitness levels; general day at work; and even hormonal levels. Hence what you did right the last month, last week or even one day before, might not feel as good for your partner the next time you do it.

To get closer to a 9.99 out of 10 from a sexual experience, communicating openly with your partner helps; providing feedback is definitely encouraged, not to mention learning new sexual techniques through reading a book, watching an online video, or attending a workshop. Coincidentally, I believe I am the only person teaching sexual techniques in Singapore. The ladies who have attended these workshops have expressed surprise at the number of different ways to pleasure the male anatomy. Indeed, the ways one can pleasure sexually are indefinite.

So if sex is not the same as studying from the 10-year-series and there are no definitive answers, why do I get asked over and over again: Is it normal to desire/ want/ have sex X number of times a day? Is it common to do Y? What is the best way to get him or her to achieve the big 'O'?

We are all different. There is no best way. What works with person A you were intimate with might not work for person B. Even with the same person, the experience will feel different—all things being equal—on a different day.

The best way is what works for you and the person you are with. Ask, try, evaluate, then try again.

And remember: chill out. You are not sitting for an exam.

Sex and the King of Fruits

What is the relationship between sex and durians? Is there any at all?

I like to use metaphors and analogies to make sure that I get my intended message across in the most effective way in the shortest amount of time. This has a lot to do with my first career in corporate communications, where time is of the essence and clear, simple messages often work best.

When I hear of adverse reactions to male ejaculatory fluid, also known as semen, I ask follow-up questions to better understand the aversion.

"What is it about the 'cum' that you don't like?"

"Is it the taste, smell or look?"

Sometimes I find a discrepancy. There might be an assumption that because the semen looks "disgusting" to the person concerned, it will smell or taste bad. Or the fluid smells bad and so the taste should be equally horrible.

I never try to disregard or dismiss their feelings. Instead I use the analogy of a durian.

Widely known and revered in Southeast Asia as the King of fruits, the durian is distinctive for its large size, unique odour and formidable thorn-covered husk. The fruit can grow as large as 30 cm (12 inches) long and 15 cm (6 inches) in diameter, and it typically weighs one to three kg (2 to 7 lb). Its shape ranges from oblong to round, the colour of its husk green to brown, and its flesh pale yellow to red, depending on the species.

Mention durian and you evoke immediate and quite diverse reactions—from deep appreciation to intense disgust. The edible flesh emits a distinctive odour, strong and penetrating even when the husk is intact. Some people regard the durian as fragrant; others find the aroma overpowering and offensive. The odour has led to the fruit's banishment from certain hotels and most public transportation in Southeast Asia.

You would think it stops there. But then there are those who like or do not mind the aroma but detest the taste. And yet others who dislike the odour, but in reality, do not mind the taste.

The smarter ones get it immediately the moment I say, "Think of the durian."

Most times I elaborate, "Some people like the smell, but don't like the taste. Others like the smell, but not the taste. So if you haven't tried, how do you know you really don't like it?"

The "A-ha" moment shows on their face. A shift in perception takes place.

Granted, they might find the smell and taste appalling, but at the very least they would know it for themselves. And through repeated exposure, the perceived "offence" might reduce and result in greater comfort with sexual expression.

Sex: a Job or a Joy?

Is sex a job or a joy to you? Sex means many things to different people, often depending on where they are emotionally, or even the time of their life. For some, it is a chore, a duty, an obligation, simply a way to keep the harmony in a relationship. For others, it may be a way to ensure food gets put on the table. Sex may even be viewed as a strategic decision to reduce the chances of the partner seeking sex elsewhere.

For other people, sex is pure bliss. To them, sex is their way of expressing themselves; a part of their way of life as natural as breathing. Through sex, there is the merging of two bodies; it is where two souls come together, the two hearts beating as one. Cliché as this description of enmeshment might sound, this intimate emotional connection is entirely possible and highly attainable with some conscious practice—and from there, the self-consciousness becomes less apparent, until it becomes a subconscious competency.

What I would like to focus on, however, is the type of sex that is less joy, but more of an aggravation for some. There are many possible psychological reasons why one would not want sex—they're tired, depressed, stressed from work or any other kind of anxiety. Then there is also when one is literally experiencing a headache, when sex is uncomfortable, even painful, or when a woman is going through menstruation and prefers not to have sex. Then there are those who do not want sex because they do not simply feel a need or desire for it. What happens when one has little or no interest in sex most of the time? What can one do? Here are five tips:

1. **Get honest within**

   Are you giving lame excuses, or genuine reasons for not wanting sex? Is there any element of truth in it? Rather than just sweep things under the carpet, do a check-in with yourself. Be completely honest. What would make sex better for you? The difficulties you have in coping with stress, anxiety, challenges, should all be considered.

2. **Quality vs. Quantity**

   A person with low sexual drive will also want to increase the frequency of sexual activity to appease their partner. Rather than focusing on the quantity, how about also exploring the quality of it? If sex was more pleasurable, would you want to do it more often? It is not quite chicken-and-egg. It can be something that can be pursued concurrently.

3. **Examine the repercussions**

   Are you afraid of the cold shoulder you receive from your partner when you say no to sex? Have you found yourself "forcing" yourself to have sex? Or have you faked an orgasm just to get it over with? If there were no repercussions... if you were not afraid, what would you do differently? Explore that.

4. Communicate, communicate, communicate!

You really need to be communicating with your partner about what support you need—be as specific as possible. Falling silent, changing the subject, or making faces to confuse your partner is only going to prevent any authentic communication, and become counterproductive. Sexual communication is still communication. With practice, it will become easier asking for what you want in the bedroom.

5. Get professional help

There is no need to be struggling like a lone warrior. There is no glory in pain. You may wish to consider engaging a clinical sexologist or sex therapist. Sexual counselling or coaching can only make a strong relationship even more solid.

Sex should not feel like a burden, duty or chore. This statement also assumes that sex is only about penetrative sex. There are indefinite ways to engage in sexual pleasuring and enjoyment without penetration. One is limited only by the limit to one's imagination.

In this day and age, a man who doesn't bring his partner to sexual peak is called a lousy lover. This pressure to perform and be a "real man" is so intense that sometimes he has difficulties attaining his orgasm. Sex should not be about needing to prove one's manhood, outlasting your partner or denying your own pleasure.

It is perfectly normal that:

- Sometimes one of you experience an orgasm first;
- Sometimes one of you may choose <u>NOT</u> to have an orgasm;
- Sometimes one of you do not attain an orgasm;
- Or at other times both of you might not experience an orgasm.

It is all fine and perfectly normal. However, if this continues for a period of time and causes distress, it is also normal, and highly recommended, that you seek support by consulting a medical doctor, urologist, gynaecologist or a sexologist like myself.

Sex should be mutually enjoyable and pleasurable. Yes, for both of you. And it is also okay to give yourselves permission to be funny and silly. If you cannot relax with your partner in bed—making jokes, laughing at yourselves and trying new things together—then doesn't it limit the amount of enjoyment you might experience? The two of you should be relaxed, engaged, enjoying the experience and wanting more of such intimacy and joy in your lives.

SELF-LOVE

My Body in the Mirror

How many people do you know who are truly happy with their bodies?

Be honest: Are you satisfied with yours? If not, you might have a body image issue.

Body image does not just refer to aspects of our physical appearance, attractiveness and beauty. It also has to do with the mental picture you have of your own body as well as your thoughts, feelings, judgements, sensations, awareness and behaviour.

Our relationship with our bodies is ever changing—sensitive to changes in mood, environment, and physical experiences—and not usually based on facts. What we perceive of ourselves in the mirror is learned. We view our own physical attractiveness based on what is expected culturally, including from the media, our family and our peers.

Your relationship with your body does influence your behaviour, self-esteem and psyche. When we feel bad about our body, the satisfaction level with our own lives decreases. This might cause a myriad of difficulties, which may include our sexuality, careers and relationships.

How do you shift towards a more healthy and positive view of yourself?

1. **Question messages portrayed in the media**

   Many of the images of celebrities and models presented in the media have been heavily computer enhanced and airbrushed. Start questioning images depicted in the media and question why you should feel compelled to "live up" to these unrealistic standards of beauty and/or thinness.

2. **Recognise body misperception**

   Perhaps you are truly not as "fat" as you think. You might be "blind" to your own figure because of your own distortion of reality. It is important to recognise this misperception and attribute it to the disorder. Judge your size according to the opinions of people you already trust until you can trust your new and more accurate self-perceptions.

3. **Stop discriminating**

   Be conscious of the ways you are mentally discriminating against people who do not fit the norm of what is "beautiful". Work on accepting people of all sizes and shapes. This will help you appreciate your own body.

4. **Quit dieting**

   Dieting is not only unhealthy but creates mood swings and feelings of hopelessness. Instead of feeling better about yourself, you only lose your self-esteem and energy. If you feel pressure to lose weight, talk to a loved one or seek professional help.

5. Befriend your body

Recognise that you do not have to compare yourself to other people. There might be several areas of your body you cannot change. However, you can modify your beliefs and attitudes which influence the way you feel about yourself. Focus on overall health and not size.

A negative body image is a serious problem and has damaging effects on one's self-esteem. When you can smile back at your reflection in the mirror, you are well on your way to self-love and respect. Love and enjoy the person inside.

Here are some questions men have asked me.

Q *Does body hair get in the way of better sex?*

A Your body hair is what makes you a man. Acceptance of each other does not just include the idiosyncrasies, but also extends to each other's bodies.

Q *Are there any advantages to either waxing my pubic hair or keeping it trimmed or just keeping it natural?*

A The only thing about unshaven pubic hair is that strands may get caught in her mouth when she is giving you a blow job. Some women do not like the sight of hair and prefer it clean. So it may boil down to whether the guy concerned wants a blow job! Most men would prefer to keep it natural and would opt for trimming rather than shaving or waxing. In our climate where heat and moisture can get trapped more easily, it is best to wash up so there isn't any bad smell anyway.

Q *Will it be uncomfortable for the girl if you've trimmed that area and the hair's growing back and it's prickly for instance?*

A It is probably more prickly and uncomfortable for the male than female, since he is actually the one feeling it. The after effects of waxing, where the pubic hair is growing out again, takes getting used to.

Q *Or do women prefer it to be smooth?*

A If they have a choice, they might prefer it smoother for the simple reason of not having pubic hair ending up in their mouth. However again, it may come down to personal preference. Trimming that area will help give the illusion of length at least, so that's a reason to at least trim, yeah?

Q *When I trim my pubic hair, it becomes itchy, how do I avoid having this happen?*

A It is normal to feel itching around your crotch area after shaving. However, you should not scratch as it will trigger more irritation and make matters worse. Do not use talc, alcohol or aftershave. Your scrotum has very delicate skin. Instead, you may want to first soak in the shower before shaving, lather with a sensitive skin formula, before shaving in upward strokes with a sharp blade. Avoid repeat strokes in the same area to reduce irritations.

You are Truly Beautiful
Finding, accepting and embracing your inner sexy

If I had a million dollars each time I was asked how a single lady can appear sexier to the opposite gender, I would be rich.

But, there are several flaws inherent to this question.

First of all, why would you feel the **need** to appear sexier? You are essentially saying there is something fundamentally wrong—or not good enough, currently—with you. Are you being "sexy" for others, or for yourself? It is almost as if the reason why you haven't met your mate is because there is something wrong with you—not what you are doing.

Next off, why **appear** sexier? I take great offense with the word "appear". Are you saying you are not sexy enough and need to *fake* sexy? Whatever happened to identifying with your inner beauty or vixen and being sexy from inside out?

Third, what is this fixation with **sexier**? Are you feeling the pressure to act up because of societal expectations of a single person? Are you being influenced by media portrayals of what it means to be desirable? The assumption is that appearing sexier is what will attract the opposite gender. Sure it works sometimes, but would it work to attract the kind of guy you want?

Fourth, who went out and decided what **sexy** was for the rest of us? What sexy means to me is very different from what sexy means to you. By trying to "appear sexy", you are assuming so many things, including that there is only one kind of sexy. And by that it means what? For ladies, could it be short skirts, high heels, natural make-up, clear complexion, long hair, dangling earrings, not forgetting gigantic boobs? For men, maybe it is a fancy car, a fancier career and a body to match?

And so, what happens then? So what if you are not sexy in the way the world says you ought to be? Does that make you a failure? A social outcast? A reject? Who exactly decides?

I would instead rephrase the question because it is so misleading on so many levels. So, the real question should be, as stated above: How can I be more attractive?

Note how I removed "appear" and replaced "sexy". Also realise that I eliminated the words "for the opposite gender", because really, what is the fun in being sexy, attractive, etc. for the sake of others? How about for **your** sake instead?

The answer to "How can I be more attractive?" **has** to be this:

To be a more attractive person, I have to BE all that I am meant to be.

In actionable terms: do inner work. Go deep within. Find out, exactly, what the true identity of this person you are, is.

The more you learn about yourself, what you stand for, and what is important to you, the more you come into your "being" or power. You can only be a wonderful lover or attractive partner when you are a wonderful and attractive person yourself.

You **are** wonderful and attractive. You just don't believe it. It is only you who doubts that you have this "star" quality.

Yet it is easy to see the potential and the magnificence in you.

It is rare that I come across somebody that I do not find attractive. It is because my definition of attractive is deeper than the skin surface. I look within. I dig. And I often find the treasure inside: the essence of the person; the substance; and what the person is truly made of.

It is unshakable, irremovable, irreplaceable and becomes only more beautiful with time and age. This is the space I hold for my clients and you alike. You are truly beautiful.

Masturbation is Self-love

Mention the word "masturbation" and what do you think of? While masturbation means different things to different people, it is one of the most misunderstood subjects in the world as it is enshrined in mystery and secrecy because of the simple reason that we speak so little about it. Masturbation may evoke massive levels of guilt and shame, as many of us were told from when we were young not to touch ourselves "down there".

You might be scowling as you read this, but do you ever stop to recognise the tremendous good that can be found in this solo-sex activity we often perform quietly, quickly, and secretly? Also known as self-pleasuring, solo sex or self-love, masturbation is 100% safe sex, relieves depression and leads to a higher sense of self-esteem amongst many other benefits.

Females masturbate too, of course. Here, however, I have included some of the most frequently asked questions on masturbation by men, and my answers:

Q *Is masturbation bad for you?*
A All human beings are born sexual and there is no limit placed on the frequency of sexual encounters humans can engage in, including masturbation (which is a good thing). Masturbation is perfectly healthy and an important part of sexual health. Like all sex, masturbation is related to

our physical, emotional, psychological, social, and even spiritual state. Be aware of your body—watch for signs of soreness or sensitivity, and slow down if needed. If your masturbation is causing you continued distress, pain, or feels compulsive, you might want to talk to a qualified sexologist.

Q *Does frequent masturbation cause premature ejaculation?*

A For most men, their earliest sexual experiences are with masturbation, done secretly and quickly for fear of being found out. It is often believed that such early experience actually condition some men's sexual response to a pattern of rapid ejaculation. In reality, masturbation is one of the best ways for men to learn about their bodies and develop confidence about their ejaculatory control in a pressure-free environment. Using lubricant, slowing down on the stroking action when you masturbate and letting yourself enjoy the sensations more are all part of the learning process. So stroke away and take your time.

Q *Should I masturbate before sex to last longer the second time?*

A The real question appears to be about lasting longer. To last longer, you can learn the stop-start technique by yourself, which is essentially slowing down before reaching the point-of-no-return. Breathing more deeply, being more present, and engaging in more foreplay will all help you to last longer. Masturbating beforehand can actually reduce your own pleasure. There is nothing wrong in masturbating early in the day or as many times as your body desires.

Q *Will I run out of sperm if I ejaculate too many times in a day?*

A There is no limit to the amount of sperm that a man's body produces. If you ejaculate several times in a row, while you may have less sperm in each subsequent ejaculation, it will return to normal levels within a day. Doctors actually remind men to ejaculate frequently to help keep the prostate gland healthy. So rest assured, you can have all the orgasms you want without your sperm ever running out. In fact, you can learn to have an orgasm without ejaculation, but that is another subject.

Q *Is it normal to masturbate after marriage?*

A Many men and women continue to masturbate when they are in a relationship, even those who are married. It does not imply that there is something wrong in the relationship. Some of the reasons married people still continue to masturbate include using it to release stress, not wanting to go through the whole process of sex, as a quick energiser, stress reliever or when the partner is not available.

Q *Is it possible to be addicted to masturbation? When is masturbation too much?*

A We are rarely educated about the importance and positive effects of self pleasure. Masturbation is safe sex and touching ourselves feels good. Different people have different sexual drives and your expression of it does not hurt anyone. However if your masturbation frequency does interfere with your daily life such that you are unable carry out what you wish to do, then you may wish to work with a counsellor or therapist. Otherwise, I would not worry about it.

Q *My foreskin opening becomes red and swollen after I masturbate. Why does this happen?*

A You are describing the head of the penis which is actually only covered by a very thin mucous membrane—it's thinner than it looks and is very sensitive. It is usually protected from friction or abrasion because of your foreskin covering it. When you masturbate, the head is exposed and the fiction can cause some reaction. The head of the penis may also be sensitive because you have ejaculated. I am not sure how long the head of your penis remains red and swollen. You also did not mention if you were in pain. If you are having any pain, it's a good idea to check with a medical doctor.

Q *I have low penile sensitivity. What can I do?*

A You are the expert of your body. Why do you think this is happening? Are you circumcised? Have you been taking any drugs that might be inhibiting your sexual desire and sensation? I am taking a stab in the dark with regards to your question when I say this: Could it have anything to do with the way you are masturbating? Most men masturbate using just their hand and nothing else. Always use lubricant when masturbating. It will feel smoother and more pleasurable as you slide your hand up and down the length of your penis, consequently causing you to reduce the grip you have on your penis.

As Woody Allen famously said, "Don't knock masturbation— it's sex with someone I love". Masturbation is a great way to learn about your own body, including ejaculatory control and mastering your orgasm potential. Let go of the guilt.

Female Readers Ask About Masturbation

In the previous chapter Masturbation is Self-love, I tackled men's most commonly asked questions about masturbation. Here are the answers to questions from female readers.

Q *I'm married and am a mother to a nine-year-old. I discovered self-loving in my early thirties and have been secretly indulging in it pretty often. I do look at pornography and even use a sex toy to make it more exciting. But after the euphoria fades, my desperate actions make me feel more ashamed. I know that there is nothing wrong with it, but how much of a good thing is too much? I've tried to stop but always end up doing it again.*

A It is wonderful that you are able to express your sexuality through self-love. Masturbation is perfectly healthy and an important part of sexual health. A good thing only becomes too much when your behaviour turns compulsive (i.e. you cannot stop yourself and have difficulty in carrying out your daily routine). We certainly don't worry about eating too much chocolate—our body knows when the indulgence is too much. Be aware of your body—watch for signs of soreness or sensitivity, and slow down if needed. I would explore the reasons why you are feeling ashamed after self-pleasuring and where the guilt stems from. I say, embrace and enjoy!

Q *I'm thinking of buying a new sex toy and am pretty confused about all these different types and materials. Dildos, dongs, lay-ons, balls and beads. Phthalate-free, silicon, glass and stainless steel. Where do I start?*

A Indeed, there is a mind-boggling range of sex toys to navigate when it comes to deciding on your first sex toy. There are actually many sex toys designed for women on the market. Most women I have met do not want gigantic phallic-looking toys and actually find them intimidating. Instead, they prefer smaller vibrators that are discreet and beautifully-designed. You will want to consider your budget, the material, colour, design as well as functionality, including types of pulsation, ability to control the volume, or if it is waterproof. You can visit my website under "Reviews" to compare some of the sex toys I have previously reviewed.

Q *I reach orgasm much easier during masturbation than during sex. Does masturbating make it more difficult for me to climax during sex?*

A Both men and women generally find it easier to attain orgasm during masturbation. This is because they touch themselves or use an object with the exact angle or pressure that brings them over the edge quickly. Also, they tend to be more relaxed when by themselves—experience less performance anxiety, or have no fear of hurting their partner's feelings. Masturbation does not make it more difficult for you to climax during sex. The reverse is actually true—learning and knowing more about your body—including what type of touch you prefer—is going to help you orgasm more easily in all situations. Go ahead and communicate your preferences to your partner so sex can only get better!

Q *During masturbation, I do things alone that I am not comfortable doing with my husband. The very act of doing something naughty or dirty just gives me such a high. Should I try to introduce some of it into our lovemaking or just keep private things private?*

A The fact that you are wondering whether you should introduce some of what is "naughty" or "dirty" to you in the bedroom is telling me that you should think about sharing at least some with your husband. They turn you on and your honesty in sharing something that has been in your mind for some time may well encourage him to share what turns him on as well. It is important to differentiate what we fantasise about with reality—and just because we think about something doesn't mean we want them fulfilled. Being able to discuss your fantasies can help you decide if there are some, or none, of them which you would like to play out in real life with your husband.

SEX SMARTS

Sex Ed

An extract from my letter to *The Straits Times* Forum Page in 2010 on the state of sexuality education in Singapore.

There have been media reports of more girls reaching puberty early. What this means is that our youth, possibly also the boys, are maturing faster physically even if they might not be mentally ready for sex.

Our world is more complex than before. Sex is romanticised and women are glamorised as sexual objects so much so that this is their reality. Social media like Facebook and YouTube have changed the way our youth make friends, date and learn. Who knows what lurks in the darkest corners of the Internet?

How do we protect our young people from low self-esteem, chronic moodiness, depression, unplanned pregnancies, domestic violence, rape, substance abuse, STIs, AIDS, self-mutilation, eating disorders, and the like? If information is power and knowledge is king, why are we as a society so fearful of providing accurate and factual sexual information to our youth?

We may want to protect our youth by teaching them to postpone acting on their sexual feelings until they are adults. In reality, we might in fact be retarding their development, which opens them up to a whole new host of difficulties. In not allowing our youth to make their own emotional and sexual decisions in adolescence, it interferes with their ability to make sound, safe and independent decisions throughout their lives.

We have to be careful not to bombard our youth with negative messages of sex being a reproductive hazard, the dangers of STIs and pregnancy sets them for a life in which they don't think about sexuality from a pleasure perspective at all. This can result in a lifelong inability to seek out sexual satisfaction and pleasure within intimate relationships.

Our young people need the skills to make safe and healthy decisions not only about sexual intercourse and contraceptive use, but about communication, relationships, diversity, and countless other issues that are related to sexuality.

Parents should let their children attend Health Promotion Board's compulsory sexuality programme. Think thrice before you opt out.

- Are you able to provide the same accurate and factual sexuality education?
- How would my child feel about being taken out of class while the rest of the class goes ahead?
- Remember, your child is going to get the same information afterwards from their classmates—distorted no less. Your child might also be teased for having over-protective parents.

Hence you might actually be doing more damage than good. You can still discuss what was taught in school as well as express your sexual views and values at home.

The phenomenon of early puberty is not new. Parents have previously expressed their desire to communicate more openly about sexuality with their teenager.

***

First of all, I do not agree that you can call a sex education programme comprehensive IF it is only about abstinence.

Secondly, an abstinence-only programme has been proven not to work/fail miserably. Teenage pregnancy actually increased not decreased during George Bush's presidency when his government pumped in record amounts of money to promote abstinence. Many sexologists I know of, and for whom I have great respect, have spoken out again and again against abstinence-only education. I can but I rather not be doing your research on this point.

Thirdly, by saying that we need to teach "teenagers to respect themselves, and build their self-esteem and assertiveness so that they do not conform to peer pressure/a partner's pressure to have sex", you are assuming that these are the reasons they are having sex.

Young people are having sex because they are choosing to have sex. They may not have the access to or awareness or knowledge about STI, HIV, safer sex but this is because they do not know what they do not know. They own their bodies. If there was more information, knowledge and meaningful conversations of what sex is and the personal consequences they are making, they can make more informed decisions.

But the decision is theirs to make, not for their parents, friends or the government to tell them. If anything, teenagers do not like being told what to do/not to do.

Fourthly, we are sexual beings. There is nothing wrong wanting to be sexual and being sexual (note: this can mean being sexual alone, by choice). Sexual right is a human right, including the right to use contraception, the right to have access to information, and the right to be taught this information.

The real question is when are we going to start talking to our teenagers the way they deserve to be spoken to? When are we going to stop talking down to them and telling them how they should lead their lives? We live in a globalised world with an MTV generation. We are spending more years in school. People are getting married later. And as teenagers with hormonal overdrive, you want to tell them what—don't be sexual? Our sexuality is not a on-off button that we can turn on at a convenient time preferably after marriage. If anything, I see lots of people who are physically and sexually shut down and having major sexual difficulties because of negative sexual messages.

Sweeping this issue of comprehensive sexuality education under the carpet and ignoring that Asians are just as sexual as our western counterparts in the name of different "culture" is highly simplistic, moralistic and going to be ineffective. Am I surprised by the rising pregnancies and STIs? No. Honest dialogues and a comprehensive sex ed programme are overdue. If you want me to agree with you that abstinence is the way to go, I cannot.

Heterosexuals: Come On Out

You might have come across the term "coming out". What does it mean?

It is a figure of speech used by the lesbian, gay, bisexual and transgender (LGBT) community in disclosing their sexual orientation and/or gender identity. Also referred to as "coming out of the closet", the beginning of this process is acceptance of oneself. Following this, openness may occur with family, friends, co-workers, the community in which one lives, etc. This is a life-long process. One can "come out" similarly or in a different manner to various individuals or groups at different times.

If you are a heterosexual, "coming out" might seem like an alien concept. Below is a tongue-in-cheek questionnaire developed by Martin Rochlin, PhD, in 1977, designed to illustrate the implicit heterosexism in these same questions asked of lesbians and gays.

Heterosexism is the belief that everyone is, or should be, heterosexual. It is the belief that rights and privileges should only go to heterosexuals and that any other sexual or romantic orientation either doesn't exist and/or is inferior to heterosexuality. Gays and lesbians experience these questions in the same way a heterosexual would.

Questions for Heterosexuals
(Developed by Martin Rochlin, PhD, 1977)

1. What do you think caused your heterosexuality?
2. When and how did you first decide you were a heterosexual?
3. Is it possible your heterosexuality is just a phase you may grow out of?
4. Is it possible your heterosexuality stems from a neurotic fear of others of the same sex?
5. Isn't it possible that all you need is a good gay lover?
6. Heterosexuals have histories of failures in gay relationships. Do you think you may have turned to heterosexuality out of fear of rejection?
7. If you've never slept with a person of the same sex, how do you know you wouldn't prefer that?
8. If heterosexuality is normal, why are a disproportionate number of mental patients heterosexual?
9. To whom have you disclosed your heterosexual tendencies? How did they react?
10. Your heterosexuality doesn't offend me as long as you don't try to force it on me. Why do you people feel compelled to seduce others into your sexual orientation?
11. If you choose to nurture children, would you want them to be heterosexual, knowing the problems they would face?
12. The great majority of child molesters are heterosexuals. Do you really consider it safe to expose your children to heterosexual teachers?

13. Why do you insist on being so obvious, and making a public spectacle of your heterosexuality? Can't you just be what you are and keep it quiet?

14. How can you ever hope to become a whole person if you limit yourself to a compulsive, exclusive heterosexual object choice and remain unwilling to explore and develop your normal, natural, healthy, God-given homosexual potential?

15. Heterosexuals are noted for assigning themselves and each other to narrowly restricted, stereotyped sex-roles. Why do you cling to such unhealthy role-playing?

16. Why do heterosexuals place so much emphasis on sex?

17. With all the societal support marriage receives, the divorce rate is spiraling. Why are there so few stable relationships among heterosexuals?

18. How could the human race survive if everyone were heterosexual, considering the menace of overpopulation?

19. There seem to be very few happy heterosexuals. Techniques have been developed with which you might be able to change if you really want to. Have you considered aversion therapy?

20. Do heterosexuals hate and/or distrust others of their own sex? Is that what makes them heterosexual?

If somebody you know is coming out to you, be neutral, non-judgemental and compassionate. We are all taught, from our youth onwards, to treat everyone with respect and this applies regardless of one's sexual orientation or gender identity.

Street Smart or Sex Smart?

So, how did you select your secondary school after your PSLE (Primary School Leaving Examinations)? How did you decide what career to pursue? Before any major purchase, what would you do before making the final choice?

Of course, you must have conducted some form of research into all kinds of things—from the best places for luxury bargains, which degree to pursue, what career prospects exist, to which type of housing is affordable. This research might have taken the form of asking trusted friends, seeking advice from family members, or even surfing the Internet, to help you make all sorts of decisions.

Now to my point—why don't we take that care when it comes to sex and sexuality? What exactly do you know about sex and sexuality? Surely, this topic deserves some of your attention, considering how uninformed or bad decisions can be detrimental to your well-being? How about learning what you should know so you can at least go out and get the necessary information?

Many women believe that they know enough about sex and sexuality. Why wouldn't they? They've dated, they know what's going on, they're street smart and noone will take advantage of them. They know how to look after themselves, right?

Sex and sexuality are two distinct terms, which are often thought, incorrectly, to have the same meaning. While sex is an activity usually involving sexual intercourse between two persons, sexuality is a much broader term. Sexuality education is a lifelong process of acquiring information and forming the attitudes, beliefs and values of one's sexuality. It encompasses sexual development, sexual and reproductive health, interpersonal relationships, affection, intimacy, body image and gender roles.

Contrary to popular belief, sexuality education, HIV or STI prevention, and adolescent sexual education programmes do not encourage the early start of sexual intercourse, the frequency of intercourse, or even an increase in the number of sexual partners among the young. Instead, understanding sexuality can actually delay the onset of intercourse, reduce the frequency of intercourse, reduce the number of sexual partners, and increase condom or contraceptive use.

These are some things a sexually informed person ought to know:

- Sexual development and reproduction—the physical and emotional changes associated with puberty and sexual reproduction, including fertilisation and conception.
- HIV/STI and safer sex practices—information on HIV/ STI and modes of transmission, how to prevent yourself and your loved ones from these infections as well as where to go for medical advice if you ever contract these infections.
- Contraception and birth control—what contraceptives are available, how they work, how people use them,

how to decide what to use or not, and how they can
be obtained.
- Relationships—what kinds of relationships there are,
love and commitment, marriage and partnership, the
importance of self-esteem and communication skills in a
relationship and the law relating to sexual behaviours and
relationships as well as the range of religious and cultural
views on sex, sexuality and sexual diversity.

Some good web resources include:
- Scarleteen (http://www.scarleteen.com)
- WebMD (http://www.webmd.com/sex-relationships/
default.htm)
- HPB Sexual Health (http://tinyurl.com/pxtmmwm)

I'd like you to really think about it, and answer (to yourself),
honestly: What do you *really* know about the topics above?
Are you making good decisions about your sexual health? Are
you well-informed about all these issues? And, if not, what
can you do about it? Can you be not just street smart, but sex
smart as well?

C is for Condom

Some of the sexuality education workshops I run contain a safer sex component where I demonstrate how ladies can put on a condom for their partners. Once, a lady asked candidly why the demonstration was relevant to her since all her sexual partners in the past would put on the condom themselves.

Indeed, why should we learn to put on a condom, or for that matter—ride a bicycle, change a flat tire or anything for ourselves—if the people around us will always do these things for us? What if, one day, she was to meet a man who resisted wearing a condom and would only use one if she were to put it on? Would she know how to since she has never had to do it?

Realising that it was not true that their sexual partner always has their welfare at heart, the class really sat up and paid attention for they recognised that it was their safety that could be compromised. It is your body and here are some essentials any woman should know:

How to put a condom on:
- Make sure you have a good quality condom that is new, and which has at least six months left until the expiration date. A condom which has been exposed to temperatures that are too warm or cold is not recommended, such as those having been in pockets, the car, or a wallet.

- Check to see you are unrolling the condom the right direction over an erect penis.
- Pinch the tip of the condom while you unroll the condom down to the base of his penis.
- When removing a condom, hold the base as you pull the condom off before throwing it into the bin (not the toilet bowl). Never use condoms twice.

What should you say when you want him to don a condom but he puts up all kinds of protests? Realise that a firm "No" should suffice—no further explanation is needed. You do not need to be tripping over yourself or bending over backwards to please him. You want him to respect you as an individual and as a person, and compromising your health and well-being may lead him to lose respect for you. Surely, you want to be true to yourself and be able to hold your head up high, throughout the entire relationship—however it turns out.

One tip to rebut his excuses is to use the keywords in his sentence, and incorporate them into your response. It shows him that you are acknowledging him, without being aggressive at all. Here are some examples:

If he says: *"Condoms ruin the mood."*
Your possible reply: *"Having unsafe sex ruins my mood. I cannot have sex when I don't feel protected."*

If his excuse is: *"I cannot enjoy sex with a condom."*
Your possible reply: *"The protection will allow me to enjoy sex."*

If he says: *"If you really love me, you should trust me."*
Your possible reply: *"It is because I love you that I want to be sure we're both protected."*

If he complains: *"I can't feel anything when I'm wearing a condom."*
Your possible reply: *"Have you tried using a thinner condom that can provide better sensations?"*

If he says: *"Condoms don't work anyway. Why bother?"*
Your possible reply: *"Condoms used correctly are 98% effective."*

If his excuse is: *"Wearing a condom is uncomfortable."*
Your possible reply: *"Not wearing a condom is not an option for me. Have you tried using this brand?"* (Suggest a different brand or size. Consider different condom types besides latex condoms.)

If he persists, repeat what you just said. Here are other ways to say no:

I mean it.
I said, "No."
I said, "Cut it out."
I asked you to ____.
I asked you not to ____.
I want you to ____.
I really would like you to ____.

Some men will continue trying to worm their way out of putting on a condom if they can. His lack of respect about what you need to feel safe and consideration for your well-being may be a tell-tale sign of the type of person he is and where the relationship might be headed. Be smart, be alert, and please, be safe. There is only one of you.

Here are some questions men have asked me.

Q *What are the things to look out for when buying a condom?*

A Size of condom for fit; and safety precautions including checking if the box is sealed and that the expiry date is at least six months from the purchase date. Most quality brands do indicate the size of the condom on the box.

Q *How do you know if you're a large, medium or small?*

A Measure. Besides putting on the condom properly, the effectiveness of a condom and the sexual pleasure possible has also to do with getting the right fit.

Q *How should guys measure themselves?*

A **Length**. You can use a ruler to measure your erect penis. This means the side furthest from your testicles, to the tip of your shaft. You will find it easiest holding the ruler against the base of your penis. While it is true that condoms can stretch to many times their normal size, men with larger penises may experience condom breakage more frequently than men with typical- or smaller-sized penises. In addition, if a condom is too short, some STIs could be transmitted between the exposed part of the penis and the partner.

Girth. Wrap a tape measure around your penis at its base to measure the girth or thickness. If your girth is above average, a standard-sized condom might feel uncomfortably tight and the larger-sized condoms could be appropriate for you.

Having some curvature doesn't mean you need a special kind of condom. Latex is very thin and flexible, so any kind of condom will work just as well for men with curvature as they will for men without. These two dimensions will give you a better idea of what type of condoms you should be getting. Most quality condom brands do indicate the size of the condom on the box.

Q *What are the dangers of picking a condom that's the wrong fit?*

A A poorly-fitting condom can undermine its effectiveness in preventing STIs and pregnancy, as well as interfere with the pleasure and sensations for both partners during sex. Different condom manufacturers use slightly different measurements and have a number of shapes available, so you may want to try different condoms until you find one which is most comfortable for you.

Q *Do the ribbed condoms really enhance sensation?*

A Yes ribbed condoms can enhance sensations. Try to see if she likes the experience as well.

Q *Any precautions to note when using a condom?*

A Condoms feel better and are less likely to fail when you put them on correctly. With perfect use, condoms are highly effective, around 98%.

- Check for latex allergic. There are other types of condoms on the market which are for those allergic to latex. For instance, Durex Avanti is for those allergic to latex.

- Extra thick condoms really don't provide any extra protection. So using regular or ultra thin is just fine.

- Never use two condom as the chance of breakage actually increases.

- A lot of guys tend to put their condoms in their pockets or wallet or the glove compartment in their car out of convenience. They do not always realise that the heat from the vehicle or wallet can disintegrate the condom and compromise the quality of the condom. Condoms kept in pockets or wallets may be more likely to tear due to the fiction or back and fro rubbing of the condom in the packaging from sitting and walking.

Q *Can you tell me more about flavoured condoms. The flavour is located on the outside to reduce the risk of an STI being transmitted orally, but if oral sex is performed on a condom is there not a risk of the condom breaking or tearing if it catches on a girl's tooth accidentally? Also once the flavour runs out is it left with the regular latex?*

A Some STIs can be passed on orally, so it's a good idea to put on a condom for oral sex. Flavoured condoms would be the same strength as well as have gone through the same rigorous testing as the normal condoms so you shouldn't worry about it at all. There is a chance of the condom breaking or tearing if the girl is actually biting or chewing on the condom as part of the oral sex. It is a good idea to change the condom before vaginal penetration. In addition, flavoured condoms that contain sugar could throw off the pH level inside of a girl's vagina (leading to yeast infections), so make sure they are sugar-free!

Q *Can I use the condom in water?*

A Condoms are perfectly safe to use in water. Having sex in water can be tricky because the lubrication (whether vaginal or from the condom) tends to get rinsed away. Without enough lubrication, the friction can cause the condom to break. Therefore you may wish to use silicon-based lubricants which do not rinse away as easily, and yet are perfectly safe when used with latex. It is easier to apply it outside of water.

Q *Why do I often have UTI (urinary tract infection) almost everytime after having sex? Is it something to do with the condom ?*

A One reason why women may get repeated infections is because previous infections can damage the internal lining of the bladder, called the mucosa, which may necessitate longer courses of antibiotic treatment. The mucosa is an essential barrier to the bacteria that normally enter the bladder. You may consider seeing a urologist to figure out exactly what's going on with you. The urologist may perform a cystoscopy, to rule out interstitial cystitis, and/ or put you on prophylactic or post-intercourse antibiotics or some other treatment. Prevention strategies include: drinking lots of water; emptying your bladder before and after sex; boosting your immune system by eating plenty of fruits and vegetables rich in antioxidants, vitamins and fibre; exercising; refraining from or quitting smoking; and getting enough sleep. Frequent UTIs are not normal and being vigilant can be key to managing frequent infections.

Oral Sex is Not Always Safe Sex

I have run a blow job workshop for ladies—52 times to date (as at time of writing) actually. During the workshop *Funtastic Fellatio*, whenever I state that oral sex is not safe sex, I inadvertently get raised eyebrows or questioning looks from the female participants.

A few honest ones would admit that they never knew about this fact. They would insist on condom use during sexual penetration, but would also "go down" on the guy without a condom. They assumed that one only catches STIs through penetrative sex—perhaps due to the widespread advocacy of condom usage.

I should not be surprised because until I received extensive training towards becoming a sexologist, I actually knew very little about safer sex practices other than the need to put on a condom during sex. I assumed I should have known better and just mistakenly thought other women were smarter and wiser.

Our ignorance may result in dire repercussions to our health. A study released by Ohio State University in 2011 stated that over the last 20 years, there has been a surge in cases of oral cancer linked directly to the human papillomavirus, or HPV, by about 58%. By 2020, the virus which mostly affects men is expected to become more common than HPV-caused cervical cancer. A similar study conducted by Johns

Hopkins University in 2007 also found HPV to be a stronger risk factor for throat cancer than tobacco or alcohol use. In case you didn't know, there are several STIs which have no cure, besides HIV—HPV and herpes being just two of them.

Modern-day women should know about safer sex practices and the extent of sexual risk they are exposing themselves to, but they do not. Therefore, I want to highlight the different types of sexually behaviour one engages in and the risk factors.

Guidelines for risk management

Safe	Possibly Safe
Massage	French kissing
Hugging	Anal intercourse with
Mutual masturbation (touching your own genitals)	condom
	Vaginal intercourse with
	condom
Dry kissing	Fisting with glove
Voyeurism, exhibitionism	Cunninglingus with latex
Phone/ computer sex	barrier
Sex toys (provided condoms are used if toys are shared)	Fellatio with condom
	Rimming/analingus with
	latex barrier
Bathing together	Finger fucking vaginally or anally with latex glove or cot
	Watersports (urine on unbroken skin)

Possibly Unsafe	Unsafe
Cunnilingus without a barrier	Anal intercourse without condom
Finger fucking without a barrier	Vaginal intercourse without condom
Fellatio without a condom	Blood contact
Sharing sex toys with cleaning or changing condoms in between uses	Unprotected cunnilingus during menstruation
Fisting without a glove	
Rimming/ analingus without a latex barrier	

Source: Winks, C. & Semans, A. (2002) *The Good Vibrations Guide to Sex,* 3rd edition, Cleis Press Inc, USA, p. 293.

I am not suggesting that you prefer one box of sexual activity— for instance only choosing to engage in safe sexual activity— over another for the rest of your life. I'm not encouraging you to go out and do anything you do not wish to. Instead, I am encouraging you to recognise the risks and learn how to manage those risks.

Taking care of yourself means making informed, and hopefully better, decisions for you—because you have to put yourself first. This is your body, your life, your future we are talking about. And remember, oral sex is not safe sex—a condom over the penis makes it safer, not 100% safe, but it may save your life.

Q *What are some safe oral sex practices you would recommend for a woman and her partner? [eg: don't be afraid to negotiate condom use? Dental dams?]*

A When it comes to HIV, oral sex is safer sex than vaginal or anal intercourse. But other infections, like herpes, syphilis, and hepatitis B, can be passed by oral sex. Condoms or other barriers can also be used to make oral sex even safer.

- Be prepared to talk about the risks of oral sex and why being safe is important to you. It might help to print out the list of STIs that can be transmitted through oral sex.

- Focus on the fact that safe oral is still oral sex. And that if it's something your partner likes, agreeing to do it with a condom may get him more of it.

- You may wish to use a flavoured condom or use a flavoured lubricant over a condom for inspiration.

Q *We recently did a survey amongst women and found that most women would rather give than receive oral because they felt that they smelt, looked or tasted funny down there. Would you, in your professional opinion, say that these types of attitudes are normal?*

A Yes, it is commonly expressed by the people who come to see me. I run a blow job workshop and even among those who are open to performing fellatio on their partner are some who do not know how to give good oral sex, and are also a bit disgusted by the idea of it.

Performing fellatio is a choice and personal preference. Oral sex is just something that a lot of people happen to enjoy and become more comfortable with when they're older. While oral sex can be very enjoyable, it is not the rolls royce of sexual acts, and there are other ways of producing similar pleasure. Couples who are at odds over oral sex need to give each other some room. They could also privately examine their feelings about oral sex, discuss them so as to explore and understand them.

There are various techniques to perform oral sex and there is no need for women to feel that they must take their partner's entire penis into their mouth. There is a range of ways one can perform oral sex on a man. Similarly, there are different positions couples can use for oral sex on a woman.

Q *And if yes, why do you think women are prone to feel this way?*
A This may be spawned from
- the lack of understanding and comfort about sex and expressing their sexuality;
- being overly concerned about cleanliness;
- religious beliefs; and/or
- really bad experiences with previous partners.

"This is afterall where he pees from" is a common comment. In reality the genitals of a healthy man (or woman) are actually "cleaner" than our mouths. Being put off by the taste or odour of the genitals is often more of a mental response than a physical one.

Another reason some women might not be too excited about giving men oral sex is that they think they don't have the skills to properly please a man i.e. don't know, don't want to do it. In addition, she has to contend with the fear of not being good enough. There is the fear of the unknown i.e. never done it, don't know what to expect. There is also the fear of gagging and of him ejaculating in her mouth (lack of ejaculatory control on his part).

Q *Do you think women are conditioned to feel insecure about receiving oral sex?*

A See above. It is not just that they necessarily feel insecure about doing it. They may not; they may just not like doing it or the idea of doing it. Different.

Few other things:

- On swallowing—Performing oral sex on a man or fellatio does not means that you *have* to swallow the semen if you do not wish to, and he should respect your wishes. No one should ever feel pressured or coerced in lovemaking. You can always have him ejaculate in your mouth, spit it out discreetly into a tissue or excuse yourself and wash out your mouth in the toilet. Or you can give him oral over a condom so he ejaculates inside your mouth, not into it.

- On gagging—Your gag reflex is a normal reaction that prevents the passage of anything from the throat, except during normal swallowing. To deliver more of a deep throat experience, you may approach his penis directly from top down as he lies on his back so you can get his penis further down your throat. When the tip of his penis meets the back of your throat, you should practise relaxing your throat muscles further rather than panicking. During this time, you can either hold your breath, breathing again when you come up for air, or breathe through your nose.

Sex tip: One common complaint I receive from ladies who perform fellatio on their partner is how their gag reflex is triggered when the penis hits the back of their throat. You can prevent gag reflex from happening by wrapping your fingers around the base of the penis, he will thus not be able to penetrate too deeply.

Ⓠ *What would you recommend women can do to feel more comfortable about receiving oral?*

Ⓐ You may not be comfortable with or may even dislike certain sexual acts like oral sex at the beginning, but this does not mean that your attitude will not evolve with time. We are all on the journey of life, albeit a sexual one in this instance. And our thoughts, beliefs and attitudes will evolve i.e. change over time. Things that may have seemed gross before, you may see in a different light once you are more comfortable with yourself or as you enter into a stable loving relationship and wish to better pleasure your partner . Remain open-minded and try to seek out answers for yourself even if tentatively, instead of relying on only hearsay. If you feel distressed about your sexuality and how it compares against other people, you may wish to seek professional support.

Q *Is swallowing sperm safe/hygienic?*

A Swallowing semen is not a negative or perverse act. Sexual norms vary from person to person. Semen and sperm are digested with all your other food in your stomach if swallowed. A woman cannot get pregnant from swallowing sperm. If your sexual partner has no STIs, it's perfectly safe. It's 95% water anyway as well as a highly concentrated source of protein, minerals, natural sugars and other nutrients which doesn't contain any harmful chemicals. On that note, you should always practise safe sex and get tested often.

Q *How can a man best use his tongue to bring a woman to orgasm? What are some techniques he can try?*

A Our fingers are hard, dry and possibly chafing. On the other hand, your tongue is warm and moist, hence probably superior to the penis in giving her an orgasm. Also it is easier for most women to achieve clitoral rather than vaginal orgasms, and oral sex is very effective in triggering such orgasms.

- Start slowly—many women like it when their partner takes his time and appreciates her body. Try dragging your tongue from her belly down to her vagina, letting your tongue brush against her labia, then gently sucking the tip just inside the vagina. You can also lick her vagina from the vaginal opening all the way to her clitoris. The best trigger for most women is the clitoris. It's the small nub of flesh outside and to the front of the vagina.

- Move your tongue from her inner lips to her outer labia. Suck her lips into your mouth and run your tongue over them. Be sure to give the other side the same amount of attention. Vary the pressure and speed of your licks to help maximise the pleasure.

- Suck her clitoris into your mouth as her pleasure becomes more intense, continually sucking and flicking it with your tongue. Start out slow and work up to your speed. Enjoy her tastes and smells, get to know every part of her vulva. While you're going, you can also try massaging her nipples and see if she likes it. The double stimulation and consistent pressure on her clitoris might just push her over the edge to pure ecstasy.

Sexual Consent

So what exactly is consent when it comes to sex?

According to Scarleteen, a popular sexuality resource website for young people, consent is:

- Voluntary: Not coerced.
- Sober: A person who is intoxicated cannot legally give consent.
- A process: Asked for at every step of the way.
- Verbal: If you want to move to the next level of sexual intimacy, just ask.
- Informed: Never implied and cannot be assumed.
- Mutual: Both people should be involved in the decision to have sex.
- Wanted: Just because you are in a relationship does not mean that you have permission to have sex with your partner, even if sexual activity has already occurred.
- Enthusiastic: The absence of a "no" doesn't mean "yes", and "maybe" is still a "no".

Indeed, Section 90 of the Penal Code in Singapore states that there is no consent (*a*) if the consent is given by a person under fear of injury or wrongful restraint to the person or to some other person; or (*b*) if the consent is given by a person who, from unsoundness of mind, mental incapacity, intoxication, or the influence of any drug or other substance, is unable to understand the nature and consequence of that to which he gives his consent.

AWARE's leaflet *What is consent?* published in 2011 cautions that consent has to be expressly given to any form of penetration. It states that rape is committed when a man penetrates a woman's vagina with his penis without her consent. Penetration of the vagina or anus with fingers or the hand, or getting a woman to give a blow job without her consent constitutes "unlawful sexual penetration", which carries the same penalty as legal rape. The penalty for both offences is imprisonment for a term of up to twenty years plus a fine or caning.

I have often been asked whether seeking consent each step of the way during a sexual encounter would break the flow of activity or dampen the intensity of the emotional connection. It would appear to be disruptive; however, I would say the reverse would be true. One should not assume any entitlement to another person's body or sexuality. The verbal articulation can reduce any second-guessing, when and where non-verbal communication cues are not clear. This respect and honesty can reassure your partner, as well as build even more trust and intimacy in the relationship, which, in turn, leads to sex being a better experience. It is normal and healthy for women to communicate their needs, wants and preferences.

Let's be clear, once again, about when No means No.

Not now means No.
Wait... means No.

I rather be alone means No.
No thanks means No.
You are not my type means No.
Silence means No.
Stop means No.
Get off me means No.

Sexual assault can be extremely traumatic. Normal reactions include fear, guilt, anger, confusion, sadness, depression and shock after the incident. Ladies do not need to go through this alone.

***

Women who persist in saying no verbally and communicating yes physically are indeed, by definition, sending mixed signals. They can confuse and frustrate men. Of course the women do not deserve to be raped (no one does) but we certainly could do better at speaking up—speaking our truth so there is absolutely no confusion whatsoever.

***

We live in an imperfect world. Our world believes that women can and should do things to prevent being victimised—and this may well be her best self-defence mechanism. This is different from criticising the way she dresses and not trusting any of her male friends.

According to AWARE's leaflet on *Reducing Risks of Sexual Assault* published in 2011 tips which pertain to the above case include:

- Be smart about alcohol. It's much easier to be a victim or predator when you're trashed.
- Consent cannot be given when someone is drunk, passed out or emotionally distressed.
- Be clear and assertive. If there is any misunderstanding, say no. Respect yourself: it is always okay to say no. It is okay to change your mind. Sex is never an obligation.
- Avoid any situation where you're not completely comfortable and don't be afraid to leave any situation that makes you feel uneasy.

Educating young people on sexuality and alcohol can be challenging. While there is no excuse for some men being lechers, a woman, on her part, has to learn how to maintain control and fend off unwanted attention, maybe even not agreeing to put herself in situations where her safety will be compromised. A young person who does not know how to drink has to learn fast, or master the art of saying no; or they will be confronted with the possibility of hook-ups that occurred when intoxicated.

Don't be afraid to say no.

GETTING REAL ABOUT SEX

Sexual Milestone

If I were to have to choose one single sexual milestone, it would have to be the day when I was told to shut up while engaged in penetrative sex with my then-husband.

My first husband is also the same man who I first had sex with. He was a gentle lover for the most part. However there were instances when I did not understand how he could have disregarded my feelings. One memory had to do with how he insisted on having penetrative sex for the first time on the eve of my 21st birthday when we had agreed previously that it would on my birthday itself. I was not particularly aroused, but rather caught unprepared for the speed in which he managed to penetrate me. I did not have an orgasm and there was no blood. I remember being sorely disappointed, asking myself, "If that was sex… what is the big fat deal about it? You mean I have been waiting my whole life for… this?"

Other inconsiderate incidents involved him dragging me through "the Strip" in Las Vegas taking photographs of him posing in front of the different hotels (not of me or us, just of *him* as evidence he had visited those places) when I was cold and feeling extremely unwell. On the same trip, I had asked him to get my medication in the overhead compartment only to have him refuse, and for me to feel progressively worse for the flight from San Francisco to Japan. And these latter two instances were during my honeymoon!

Perhaps, not unlike other married couples, sex became monotonous after a while. He would fondle my breasts, lick my nipples for a short time before penetrating me, almost always in the missionary position. A variation that he began to like was him standing and penetrating me with my legs over the edge of the bed. I did not know it then, but I was starting to get bored with sex being "touch-and-go". He was not a good kisser, did not engage in much foreplay and certainly was not open to any kind of sexual experimentation.

So I tried to do what I could within the constraints of what he did not like or want. I tried to caress what I could of his legs and his chest while he was penetrating me in the upright position. In hindsight, he did not seem receptive, but I suppose I didn't pick up on it at the time.

While I was easily orgasmic and could achieve an orgasm through penetrative sex, the duration of penetration was never long enough for me. He would "pump" into me for a few minutes before ejaculating outside my body. This is known as the withdrawal method—he would pull out and ejaculate onto my stomach because, being Catholic, he did not believe in using condoms. Consequently, I would be getting into the build up towards an orgasm, only to be left hanging as he would pull out abruptly, leaving me sexually frustrated—with no orgasm. I never asked if we should use condoms instead. I did not know how to use one. I just went along with what he decided to do because he is a man, and a man (certainly one who was eight years older than me) should know what to do more than I would.

It was probably the third time when I was, again, fondling him during penetrative sex with him standing, that he said, "Don't distract me."

"Distract?," I asked.

"Yes, I am concentrating. Don't disturb me."

I was shocked. I laid there and let him finish the "deed".

Afterwards, I asked him, "What did you mean by, 'Don't distract me'?"

Him: "You know… I am trying to concentrate…. " (Now I'm a sexologist, I realise that he was probably trying to last as long as he could without ejaculating, and this involved me lying still.)

Me: "How can you say that? So… sex is about you having your orgasm? What about me… and what I want to do?"

He apologised. But the damage was done. The pain, hurt or betrayal I felt from the incident never left me. No wonder he was all right with leaving me hanging, without getting my orgasm. It was all right as long as he had his. All right—as long as I lay there, and not "distract" him. I could well have been a "hole"—any hole, or another face, or body. It wouldn't have mattered, would it? Where was the emotional connection of lovemaking? Was what we were doing considered lovemaking? We were two people who "think" we are in love, but what we were doing did not feel loving to me at all.

I do not remember how many other times we had sex after that, and if sex did get better. But this was one of the signs that our marriage was not working. This was not THE reason I later divorced him, but it was one of the reasons.

The episode made me question what sex was supposed to be about, about what it should and could mean. It is a milestone because I knew in my gut that what was happening was gravely wrong. If this could happen to me, then what about the tens and thousands, maybe millions, of unfulfilled women told by their husbands to "lay down and not distract him". I knew better—that it was wrong and unacceptable—but did they? Would they? Where would one go to get help in the bedroom? And so the seed and curiosity about sex and sexuality, and what positive sexual expression was, was planted in me.

My question for you, dear reader, is: what would be your sexual milestone? I'd like to invite you to share your story with me just as I have shared mine. There is great power and healing in writing and sharing our stories. This is my sincere invite to you. My email address is *drmarthalee@eroscoaching. com*

Revised Sexual Terms

I was browsing through an expat magazine when I chanced upon an article entitled "Well-being and Sex". Intrigued, I read the piece, only to come upon the sexual terms: "sexual transmitted diseases", "impotence" and "frigidity". The author was obviously not a sexologist because these terms are passé.

In the same week, a client asked why I used the term STI to refer to "sexually transmitted infections" instead of STD. I have also dealt with journalists who have on occasion admitted that they were unfamiliar with the terms I used. Hence, I thought this is a good time to address how sexual terms have evolved with time.

Use "STI" not "STD"

Before the term "sexual transmitted disease" (STD) was used, all diseases related to the genitals were called "venereal disease" (VD). "Social disease" was another euphemism. In recent years, the term "sexually transmitted infections" (STIs) has been preferred as it has a broader range of meaning. A person may be infected, and may potentially infect others, without showing any signs or symptoms of disease.

Also, not all STIs are transmitted through sexual intercourse. Some STIs can be transmitted via the use of drug needles after its use by an infected person, as well as through childbirth or breastfeeding. Sexually transmitted infections have been well-known for hundreds of years.

"Infection" is a more encompassing word in that it can also refer to a germ—be it a virus, bacterium or parasite that can cause disease or sickness in a person's body—whether with or without symptoms. On the other hand, a disease means that the infection is actually causing the infected person to feel sick or to notice something is wrong. For this reason, the term STI is a much broader term than STD.

Say "erectile concerns" not "impotence"

The word "impotence" is a venerable term that dates back to the 15th century. Its literal meaning is "powerlessness" and so it possesses obvious pejorative connotations. The advent of sildenafil (Viagra), which is the first oral medication approved by the USFDA (United States Food and Drug Administration) for the treatment of impotence, popularised the more recent term "erectile dysfunction" (ED).

ED is actually a common men's health problem characterised by the consistent inability to sustain an erection sufficient for sexual intercourse, or the inability to achieve ejaculation, or both. This problem can be occasional as well as periodical. The word "dysfunction" means function incorrectly or abnormally.

A sexologist, such as myself, would use the words "erectile concerns" or "erectile difficulties", as they are much gentler on the ear. Clients who come before me are distressed as it is about their condition, and there is no need to stick the knife in by telling them they are "abnormal". Most men will have erectile concerns or difficulties at some point in their life.

Who are you calling "frigid"?

In the early versions of the DSM (*The Diagnostic and Statistical Manual of Mental Disorders* published by the American Psychiatric Association), there were only two sexual dysfunctions listed: frigidity (for women) and impotence (for men). Since then, we know that there are more to the sexual difficulties a woman can experience than the failure to have vaginal orgasms.

As such, "female sexual dysfunction" is now the blanket term that replaces the word "frigidity" when referring to the inability of a woman to function adequately in terms of sexual desire, sexual arousal and/or orgasm. The term "frigidity" continues to be used but like "impotence", it is seen as an insult or derogatory term for women. As explained above, I might use the words "sexual issue", "sexual concern" or "sexual condition" when speaking with a client because we all have them from time to time.

You might say sexual terms are just words. What difference does it make? Indeed it does not make that much of a difference to the sexologist who is expected to know them all and reflect only positivity and support in session. Yet it does to the person who has that sexual condition. Also knowing and keeping up to date with the sexual terms also means you have the vocabulary to communicate clearly what you intend when you wish to.

Male Sexual Dysfunctions

During my training to be a sexologist, I was confused by the differences between PE, DE, and ED. They are, namely, premature ejaculation, delayed ejaculation and erectile dysfunction or disorder, respectively. Later, I realised it was just as confusing for the men who have sexual concerns. Hopefully, this piece will give you an idea of the four main types of male sexual dysfunctions.

1. **Ejaculation disorders**
    The most common type of ejaculation difficulty known is *premature ejaculation* (PE). It happens when a man's ejaculation occurs rapidly, much faster than what is desired by the man or his partner. PE is also known as rapid ejaculation, rapid climax, premature climax, or *early ejaculation* (EE).

    Delayed ejaculation (DE), also known as inhibited or retarded ejaculation, is when ejaculation is slow to occur. Then there is *retrograde ejaculation* which occurs when the semen from the prostate flows backwards into the bladder. This is common in males with diabetes who suffer from diabetic neuropathy (nerve damage). *Ejaculatory insufficiency* refers to insufficient semen volume, which may at times be a result of retrograde ejaculation.

2. **Erectile dysfunction**

   Erectile dysfunction is a common men's health problem
   characterised by the consistent inability to sustain an
   erection sufficient for sexual intercourse, or the inability
   to achieve ejaculation, or both. This problem can be
   occasional as well as periodical. Any diseases that affect
   blood flow such as hypertension or high blood pressure
   can cause ED.

   Who hasn't heard of the blue pill, Viagra, which can
   aid ED? If anything, we have drug companies to thank
   for popularising the term ED. And since the incidence
   of ED rises with age and humans are living longer, we
   can expect more men to have this condition. Besides
   oral medication, treatment options include mechanical
   devices and behavioural training as well as couples
   coaching.

3. **Inhibited desire disorder**

   This happens when a man has a decrease in desire
   for sex, is uninterested in sex, or is unresponsive to
   sexual stimuli. Possible causes include one's physical,
   psychological, mental or emotional state. Then there
   might be issues with his body image, intimacy or sexual
   performance. Or he could just be sexually ignorant
   about what being "horny" means, such as when a person
   is sexually "shut down" or unawakened. One should also
   rule out any kind of exhaustion, stress and/or anxiety.

4. **Orgasmic disorders**

In an orgasmic disorder, the man may not be able to achieve an orgasm and reach climax during sex. These men are usually experiencing a psychological or mental health complication which may be situational or generalised to all sexual experiences. However it could also be due to decreased penile sensation and/or other factors.

Whether the cause is physical or psychological, it is important to meet with a qualified physician to determine possible underlying medical issues. If the physical cause is ruled out, this is when you might seek support from a mental health specialist who specialises in sexual dysfunction.

Q *What can I do about premature ejaculation?*

A Premature ejaculation happens when a man ejaculates earlier than he would like to. It is also known as rapid ejaculation, rapid climax, premature climax, or early ejaculation. The average male takes less than three minutes from the time of insertion till he ejaculates. To gain greater orgasmic control, the first thing is to understand what is happening to his body when he ejaculates i.e. the functions of the prostate gland and pelvic muscles.

The next thing is gaining greater mastery of the body through exercises such as breathing, strengthening pelvic floor muscles and using the "stop and start" method. This method involves bringing yourself just before the point of no return and stopping all movement before it is too late. When the urgency to ejaculate subsides, start thrusting again, and repeat several times. By committing time and effort in doing these exercises, the majority of men are able to learn better control through therapy, without medication.

Female Sexual Dysfunctions

Many women have problems with sex at some stage in their life and it becomes more common as women get older. Having covered male sexual dysfunctions in a previous piece, let's move on to the types of female sexual problems.

Female sexual dysfunction refers to one or more of the following issues: loss of sexual desire, loss of arousal, problems with orgasm and pain during sex.

1. **Hypoactive sexual desire disorder**
    The opposite end of the spectrum from hyperactive sexual desire disorder, women with this condition avoid sexual feelings, sexual thoughts and fantasies. They do not initiate sexual activity and are not responsive to their partner's initiation of sexual activities. Causes include fatigue, hormonal changes, relationship conflict, body image issues, a history of sexual abuse, or being with an unskilled lover or partner.

2. **Sexual aversion disorder**
    Women with this condition persistently or recurrently have a phobic aversion to, and an avoidance of, sexual contact with a partner. The disturbance causes marked personal difficulty such as panic attacks (feelings of terror, faintness, nausea, palpitations). The woman

might also avoid sexual situations or potential sex partners by covert strategies.

3. **Sexual arousal disorder**

There are four types of female arousal disorders, which can occur alone or in combination with other disorders:

- **Subjective sexual arousal disorders** mean that no matter how much the woman is stimulated, whether genitally or non-genitally, and despite the occurrence of physical genital response (this means her vagina may exhibit increased lubrication), she doesn't feel aroused.
- **Genital sexual arousal disorder** means that a woman has little or no vaginal lubrication or swelling of the vulva. She might respond to non-genital stimulation, for instance an erotic video, but not to genital stimulation. This typically affects post-menopausal women.
- **Combined genital and subjective arousal disorder** refers to lacking or feeling little sexual and genital arousal.
- With **persistent genital arousal disorders,** women have excessive unwanted unprovoked genital arousal. Arousal is unrelieved by orgasms. The feelings persist for hours or days.

4. **Orgasmic disorder**

Orgasm is the moment of most intense pleasure in sexual intercourse. Women with this condition are unable to to reach a climax or orgasm. This occurs even despite high levels of subjective arousal. This is not to be confused with women who are able to attain orgasm through clitoral stimulation.

Factors associated include: distraction; performance anxiety; negative sexual beliefs or misconception; ignorance about genital sensitivity or poor technique; anxiety about letting go of control; lack of trust; history of sexual abuse or trauma; current relationship dissatisfaction; or partner-related difficulties.

5. **Vaginal pain disorders**

There are three types of vaginal pain disorders: Dyspareunia, Vaginismus and Vulvodynia.

- Dyspareunia is pain during attempted or completed vaginal penetration. This can be lifelong (primary) or acquired (secondary).
- Vaginismus is another pain disorder characterised by reflexive tightening around the vagina when vaginal entry is attempted or completed that can block entry of the penis. This is despite the woman's expressed desire for penetration and when no structural or other physical abnormalities are present. Vaginismus is actually very treatable by focusing on sex education, counselling and progressive desensitisation.
- A third pain disorder is known as vulvodynia, which

is chronic vulvar itching, burning, and pain that leads to physical, sexual and psychological distress.

When a woman experiences sexual difficulties, it is useful to seek support from a trusted medical professional such as a gynaecologist or an urologist. Sex therapists and psychotherapists may also be helpful. It is always useful to bring your partner into the discussion. Treatment varies depending on the disorder and cause. If the types of disorder overlap, more than one treatment might be required.

Six Myths about "The Magic Wand"

There is a dire lack of sexual education in Singapore; not to mention timely, accurate and positive sexual information. There are many misconceptions about the male sexual anatomy that could be preventing men and women from feeling the pleasure they deserve. It's time to set the record straight. Here are six of the most common myths, debunked:

Myth #6: The penis is dirty

There is a common misconception amongst women of the penis being unclean, smelly or downright dirty. It goes without saying that a penis, circumcised or not, will be dirty if it is not washed. Yet, in reality, the penis is an external organ, unlike the female vagina which is an internal structure, and hence more likely to be "clean", all things considered.

The penis should be washed in the bath or shower just like any other part of the body such as your armpits or your rectum. Just roll back the foreskin (if uncircumcised), wash the glans or head of the penis with soap and rinse it off with warm water.

Myth #5: Penis size is proportional to other body parts

There is a myth based on the premise that you can tell how big someone's penis is by measuring their feet, hands, or nose.

There is no scientific proof of a correlation between body part size and penis size.

It is true that there are certain genes that control the development of the limbs which also control the development of the penis in the embryonic stage. Yet, when it comes to fully-developed males, there is no absolute relation between the size of the penis and the size of the limbs or other body parts.

Myth #4: A "real man" can last all night long

This myth would have you believe that if a man is not capable of maintaining a cucumber-hard erection and performing all night, he is an incompetent lover.

Truth: Men typically reach orgasm five to ten minutes after the start of penile-vaginal intercourse, taking into account their desires and those of their partners.

A good erection is dependent on how good the blood supply is to your penis. Men who have any kind of vascular problems have high chances of their erection being affected. Smoking affects the blood vessels making them less pliable and less compliant. Avoid smoking, fatty foods and cholesterol-rich foods. Exercising and eating healthy are good things. Whatever affects the vascular system affects your erection.

Myth #3: Your penis is your most powerful sex organ

This is patently false. Your mind is your most powerful

sex organ, and your skin is your largest one! The brain programmes our sexual function, our reproductive behaviour and our sex drive. Hence, it has the potential to be our most powerful tool for accessing mind-blowing sex. This applies for both men and women.

We can use our minds to fantasise about anything— even the impossible or seemingly unattainable. Fantasies are healthy and normal as long as you can separate them from reality and accept (and sometimes appreciate) that you may not be able to fulfil them. For many, fantasies should remain that waye—fantasies—as reality creates potential for let-down.

Myth #2: You need a penis for sex to occur

There are tremendous anxieties revolving around the hardness of the penis as well as how long it stays that way. The assumption is that the man's penis is central to a woman's sexual satisfaction. Ironically, the penis is just a small part of what might be needed to have a wonderful sexual experience. Therefore, sex should be viewed as more than just penetration.

Orgasms are a very individualistic thing — there is no one correct pattern of sexual response. Whatever works, feels good, and makes you feel more alive and connected with your partner is what counts. Men will do well in focusing on making her feel important, loved and cared for, and establishing an intimate, emotional, physical, and mental connection, rather than on the tool.

Myth #1: Bigger is better

This has to be the most well-known myth, especially since guys tease or insult each other about being small in size. The penis is a symbol of male identity, sexuality and masculinity, which is why size is often fussed over among men. The notion that a larger penis equates to someone who is more masculine has, in turn, led men to think or feel that bigger is better.

The penises of Singaporean men average 3.5 to 5.9 inches in length. Most men fall somewhere in-between. Size has little to no relation to sexual performance. Sometime when a man asks what you think of his penis, he is probably insecure and actually asking for reassurance. Do your part and encourage him to appreciate his body for what it is—healthy, functioning and perfectly normal.

There you have it: six of the most common myths debunked. Take a moment, think of the penis as not an incomprehensible alien but as a magical wand promising endless hours of pleasure and ecstasy.

Q *What can I do to make my cock long and bigger? Any cream that is available?*

A See Myth #1 above, size has little to no relation to sexual performance. The vagina does not have very many nerve endings beyond the first 3cm or so. In addition, most women do not orgasm from intercourse alone. I am not aware of any proven method that is guaranteed to make a penis longer and bigger short of surgery, where there are adverse risks such as nerve damage, chronic pain, scarring, infection and erectile difficulties. Penis pumps, pills and patches can only make your penis bigger temporarily. They all work on the same principle of increasing blood flow in order to get a thicker penis. I would be wary of any body alternating devices and invariably hurting the sensitive nerves of the penis. However as long as you use your penis pump safely there is no reason not to try it if you really want to.

Vulvas and Vaginas are Pink

I didn't know I had a vulva until I went to sex school.

Don't get me wrong. I do have a vulva (pronounce "vuhl-vah") and a vagina (pronounced "vha-gine-a"). I just didn't know what they were called. I couldn't even pronounce the word penis (say "pee-nis") and called it the "pen-is".

For the longest time, I was calling the whole area "no nok" because that was what my mother said it was. For this article, I asked my parents how to spell it and realised that what I always assumed was a Teochew word is in fact Malay!

My sexuality school was the Institute for Advanced Study of Human Sexuality in San Francisco, California, USA. Sexual anatomy was one of the first things we covered. Even then I was confused about the difference between the vulva and the vagina and was too embarrassed to admit it. Needless to say, I had a lot of catching up to do.

Now, sexual anatomy is something I talk to my clients about on a daily basis. Without knowing what is "down there" and resorting to using pet names or blushing every time we refer to our private parts, just how comfortable can one be with one's sexuality, much less sexual expression? For some people, knowing and referring to our private parts by their proper names is their first step to truly owning their sexuality.

So I tell them, with a straight face, what is what and where, utilising diagrams. Some of the braver ones admit they are still confused, and seeing that they are such keen learners, I get cyber skin replicates of the male penis and female vulva out. Their eyes invariably widen. Sometimes, a glaze comes over their eyes as I launch into my speech again. I wonder whether they are absorbing the information or are overwhelmed by the surreality of the moment.

Yet I plod on. At times, I might quiz them to make sure they remember the terms correctly. Other times, I send them home with web links to navigate as home assignments.

When I first started my practice and ran previews explaining my work, I was told by well-meaning friends to skip the part about the anatomy altogether. Make it more fun, more humorous, more interactive, they suggested.

Skip anatomy? Why should I? I see myself as a sexuality educator, among the many other roles I play. Unbeknownst to my clients, talking about anatomy is actually the first step to the desensitisation process—an important one in becoming more comfortable with our sexual self and talking about it. When you talk about sex and the anatomy involved in sex using factual, scientific and accurate language, you demystify it. By calling a spade a spade, sex is no longer the elephant in the room and no longer a taboo subject. Also, this might be my only chance to provide the correct anatomical names, including the pronunciation.

Having done the anatomical talk many times now, I am better at it—more fun, more humorous, more interactive, but I am still and will still be talking about our pink bits. Say "vulva". Try "vagina". How about "penis"? Great job, class!

Slow Down, Cowboy!

When is faster not necessarily better? That's right—when we are talking about premature ejaculation or PE. PE is also known as early ejaculation or eager ejaculation. This occurs when a man ejaculates quicker or earlier than desired. It is actually a very common sexual concern.

Can you learn to last longer without resorting to medication? Yes, here are some tips:

1. **Do your Kegels**

   Kegel exercises strengthen a man's pelvic floor muscles and reinforce his neuro-bio (brain-body) connection. These are the same muscles you use to stop the flow of urine while you're urinating. You can do the squeezes (when your bladder is empty, of course) anywhere at any time—whether it is sitting at a desk, queuing, or on public transport. Kegels can help men increase their awareness of their sexual response. The Kegel squeezing can return a feeling of control when you are approaching the edge of ejaculation or "point of no return".

2. **Stop-start method**

   When you feel you are about to come during sex or masturbation, slow down, stop your hand movement, and/or think of something else. In other words, take yourself mentally out of the situation. After two or three minutes your arousal should have dropped, so you can then return to what you were doing—but take it slowly. Slow and steady will help you last longer. During intercourse, you can either slow down or withdraw altogether from your partner. It is easier to master this technique when you are by yourself masturbating.

3. **Use lube**

   You can incorporate the use of lubricant into your self-practice and further your mastery of the stop-start method. You would stimulate yourself the same way you do to the point of ejaculation and then slow down or stop until control is regained. If you should choose an oil-based lubricant, remember that it is not safe for use with condoms, and not recommended for use in vaginal penetration.

4. **Communicate**

   Discuss openly and honestly with your partner about sexual desires and needs. You might be surprised that she might not even care or be bothered about you having early ejaculation. What is a distressing condition for a man may genuinely be a non-issue for your partner. If this is a goal you wish to work on for your own sexual fulfilment, ask directly for how and in what ways you would like support. One way to take pressure off you is by agreeing to engage in other kinds of sexual activity, such as the use of sex toys or oral sex if you ejaculate early.

5. **Get professional support**

Drugs should not be regarded as the first-line treatment but *the last resort* as there may be side effects. If the above is confusing for you, you can seek professional help that doesn't rely on pharmaceuticals, preferably a trained sexologist who will coach you through the different body-mind training methods. Find somebody trained and who is comfortable talking about sexuality; who can sympathise about early ejaculation being a stressful situation, and who will be able to explain treatment methods in simple terms which you can understand. Do not assume that all doctors are equally trained and know what is best for your body.

Q *Why does my penis go soft whenever I put on a condom?*

A Anxiety, loss of sensation, and psychological resistance to wearing a condom may lead to loss of erection. It could help if your partner helps you put the condom on. You may dab a drop of water-based lubricant to the inside tip of the condom, or onto the tip of your penis for greater sensation. Some condoms (such as the ribbed ones) can actually enhance the sensation, not decrease it. Also practise masturbating with a condom to get used to the sensation.

Q *My girlfriend says cycling can damage vaginal nerves and cause a drop in sensitivity. Is that true?*

A It is been known that bike saddles can harm the sexual performance of men. A study at Yale, published in the *Journal of Sexual Medicine* in May 2006, shows that riding bikes decreases women's sexual sensation. The theory is that riding on a bike saddle places a lot of pressure on the nerves and blood vessels in the genital area—whether for man or woman. Choosing bikes which have handlebars positioned lower than the saddle may help alleviate neuropathies in females.

Q *What are some of a woman's body signals that tell a guy he's doing the right thing in bed? What signs should a guy look out for as encouragement? My research states moans, eye contact, the girl "mirroring" the guy's moves, the speed/way she moves her hips. Do you agree, and why?*

A We get turned on through our senses—seeing, feeling, touching, smelling, tasting, hearing—and through thought or fantasy. When we begin active sexual movements, we feel the flow of pleasurable feelings centering in the genitals and abdomen. The entire body is gradually flooded with warmth, generally increasing in intensity and reaching toward a peak. In both sexes, heart rate, breathing rate and flushing (if it occurs) continue to increase.

The tension in the musculature increases (in involuntary as well as voluntary muscles). During arousal, there are changes in blood pressure, pulse, and respiration rate; vasocongestion or engorgement with blood; and muscle tension. Sexual arousal is first noticeable as the blood supply to the abdomen and pelvic area increases. In the woman, sexual arousal is usually manifested by vaginal lubrication, blood engorgement, and sweating the of the vaginal walls.

In simple words: listen to the sounds she makes, the speed of her breathing, the movements of her body especially her pelvic, as well as physiological changes to her vaginal walls for signals you are doing the 'right' things in arousing her.

Q *How can I make my orgasms stronger, naturally?*

A The idea of having better orgasms isn't meant to make you feel like there is anything wrong with the orgasms you're currently having. Here are some basics:

- Breathe so your orgasm becomes more of a full body experience;
- Instead of tensing up and holding still during orgasm, move your body and let the energy spread through your body;
- Experiment and prolong the period before orgasm;
- Try to build better orgasms by doing your Kegel exercises;
- Use sex toys;
- Fantasise. Remember not to compare your orgasms with others. What works for you is good enough. There is no wrong kind of orgasm.

Clearing the Air on G-spot and Female Ejaculation

As the only certified sexologist and certified sexuality educator in Singapore, there is a wide array of sexuality questions I am asked. However, there are three questions that I continue to be asked, sometimes worded slightly differently, but essentially the same questions again and again.

They involve a mysterious spot in a woman's body, whether men have such a spot, and if women urinate during sex. Here are the answers:

Q *Does the female G-spot exist?*

A The existence of the female G-spot (named after Ernst Gräfenberg) is a controversy that rages on to this day. In early January 2010, scientists at King's College, London, declared that the G-spot does not exist, so women need not feel inadequate. Three weeks later, a group of French gynaecologists launched a counter-attack on what they called a "totalitarian" approach to female sexuality.

The G-spot is also known as the corpus spongiosum, urethral sponge and female prostate. Most easily located when the women is sexually aroused, it can often be felt by pressing on the interior front wall of the vagina with a finger or sex toy, and may produce increased pleasurable sensations when stimulated. You need to move your finger in a "come here" motion. Try also thrusting or circular movements. Ask her what feels best. The G-spot varies in size for different women. It can be about the size of a Singapore five-cent or twenty-cent coin. Rather than be caught up with whether she has a G-spot or not, it is important to remember that there is no single best way to have sex.

Q *Do men have a G-spot?*

A The male G-spot is also known as his prostate gland. It is not in the anus but can be stimulated through the rectal wall, approximately two inches in and facing toward his belly, the prostate gland is a chestnut-sized gland just below the bladder and next to the rectum. After locating his prostate, you can stimulate it to see what he enjoys— whether it is continuous but consistent pressure, flicking it or using a sex toy that vibrates against it.

Some men experience intense orgasms when their prostate glands are stimulated. Others simply enjoy a great deal of pleasure while some men don't enjoy the sensation at all. Be gentle, and as with anything take your cues from his reactions. He will let you know by his movements and body positioning what he wants.

To pleasure:
- Massage the anal sphincter. As long as the entrance to the anus is relaxed, there is no pain during penetration.
- Apply lots of water-based lubricant.

- Insert one finger or a small sex toy slowly before including two fingers if desired by your partner. You may wish to put a condom over your finger or toy for added lubrication as well as to protect against STIs.
- Experiment with different amounts of direct and consistent pressure on where the area might be. The finger needs to be moved in a "come here" motion. Try also thrusting or circular movements.

Q *Is there such a thing as the female ejaculation?*

A The female ejaculation is not a myth or circus trick. We have a bladder and paraurethral glands, both of which can and often do contain fluids. When we put pressure on those areas or the areas surrounding them, that fluid sometimes squirts out. This pressure can be due to how arousal expands things in and around our genitals, and due to actual pressure put by fingers, hands or anything else during sex.

Women who do ejaculate do so due to extensive and targeted G-spot stimulus, internal and external clitoral stimulus, or—and most commonly—a combination of the two. However, this fluid is not urine, even though it's possible some elements of urine are in the mix, or that sometimes, women ejaculating are actually urinating. Having said that, not all women ejaculate, and even for those who do, most do not ejaculate all the time.

My primary concern is that we do not label people who cannot seem to find their G-spot, man or woman, as "dysfunctional". Since there is no one single or best way to have sex, please do not ignore everything else, worry about whether one is normal and be fixated about a singular "spot". However, if you like to learn about your body, try to locate your G-spot, or learn how to ejaculate as a woman, go ahead. What is most important is that you are having fun when doing so.

Men: Orgasm Without Ejaculation is Possible

I would like to provide more information about the male orgasm and ejaculation which are sometimes regarded as one and the same thing. Some people also believe that prostate surgery, ending the possibility of ejaculation, marks the end of a male's orgasmic potential or sexual life.

In reality, male ejaculation and orgasm are two separate physiological and psychological experiences. Difficulties with ejaculation does not mean the end of a man's sexual life, but perhaps marks a different phase, where they may wish to learn to orgasm in different ways.

Indeed, men (not just those with health issues) are learning to have orgasms without ejaculation, and also, without an erection if he so chooses. They may choose to do so in order to still feel the positive effects of feeling good after an orgasm without feeling physically exhausted following their ejaculation.

When men learn to separate their orgasm from the ejaculation, they can also learn to have one or more orgasm for each ejaculation. Having multiple orgasms as a man does not mean learning to have several ejaculations in one session of sex.

In Taoist teachings on sexuality, there are explicit instructions for men on how they can experience multiple orgasms. One popular book is *The Multi-Orgasmic Man* by

Mantak Chia and Douglas Adams. Western sex researchers have also studied this experience in men and found clear physiological evidence that it occurs.

Learning to have multiple orgasms takes a fair bit of time and practice. Having a series of non-ejaculatory orgasms are not necessarily better or worse than ejaculatory ones—just different. The training may include gaining a better understanding of male sexual response, and learning to control ejaculation through the use of breath, sound, energy and touch to experience greater sexual pleasure.

Multiple orgasms defined

It is not difficult for men or women to achieve multiple orgasms. A common misconception is that they need to be consecutive. Multiple orgasms happen when someone has more than one orgasm in one sex session—breaks included. Or, a person has more than one orgasm during the course of the same sexual activity.

On why multiple orgasms are easier for women

Women are more likely to be multi-orgasmic because they do not require a refractory period immediately after an orgasm. In many cases, they are capable of attaining additional, multiple orgasms through further stimulation. The refractory period is the recovery phase after orgasm when it is physiologically impossible for a man to have additional orgasms.

Because of the hypersensitivity of the male penis immediately after ejaculation, most men would not feel a desire to continue with sexual activity. After the refractory period, a man can choose to resume sexual pleasuring if he chooses to. The recovery period can vary considerably for different men depending on their age, fitness level, and physical state that day, for instance.

On retrograde ejaculation

During ejaculation, a man experiences the semen being expelled from the testicles, and propelled by rhythmic contractions out of the urethra. In retrograde ejaculation, his semen travels backwards and into the bladder through the bladder neck instead. The most common reason for this is surgery to the prostate or the bladder neck. However, there are other reasons this happens including disruption of the nerve supply caused by diabetes, multiple sclerosis, spinal cord injury, or certain prescription medications. The orgasmic sensation may be reduced, but does *not* mean that the man does not experience an orgasm or enjoy sex even though physically it is not possible to ejaculate. Treatment for this condition would only be considered if fertility was an issue.

Focus on feeling good

Sex or orgasms should not be measured by how much ejaculate a man has, how many times he can ejaculate in a session, or even whether he can ejaculate for that matter, but by whether it *feels* good to him. If he only wants to have sex once a day, then it's *his* decision. In short, men usually just orgasm and ejaculate once because they choose to—or because that it is the only way they have learned how to orgasm.

Likewise, some women stop sexual pleasuring after experiencing their first orgasm, even though they are supposedly capable of having multiple orgasms. Sex should not be about performing or proving anything to anybody. It's about what feels *best* to us.

Desire Discrepancy

What to do when one partner wants more sex than the other

He wants more sex. You could do with less, or even without it. Or, perhaps the reverse is true: you desire more sex while he seems disinterested. This human biological sexual instinct, where an individual is interested in engaging in sex with a partner is known as the sex drive or libido. The famous pioneering psychologist Sigmund Freud refers to this as the "life energy" that animates not only the sexual instinct but also many other human drives.

You may be wondering what, exactly, influences the human sex drive. There are biological, psychological and social components. Testosterone is believed to be the biggest attributor to the biological desire for sex and its level is 20–40% higher in men than women. However, there are also social factors, like work and family, as well as internal psychological factors, such as personality type and stress levels, which should be considered.

It is very common for men to desire sex more often than their female partners. To the woman, I like to first emphasise that just because you have a lower sex drive than your partner does *not* necessarily mean there is something wrong with you. What this means is that you need to be aware of this difference and together come up with ways to fulfil both your sexual needs.

Just how can you meaningfully address this issue of desire discrepancy? Here are some tips:

1. **Get some perspective**

    Our sex drive actually changes over the course of a day, week or month, and also many times across our lifespan. Avoid making comparisons with what other people are doing. Your sexual desire is an exquisitely unique expression of individuality, and comparisons serve no one.

    Any relationship requires negotiation and compromise and that includes sex. It's unrealistic to think that either of you will get everything you want. It is more important to communicate your sexual needs and wants, and be open to dialoguing about it. Yet at the same time there is no guarantee that all the amount of thinking, feeling and talking about your relationship will result in the change you want. Once again, the key words are: negotiation and compromise.

2. **Do a self evaluation**

    A lot of times, deep down, we do have some inkling of what the problem is. You may wish to ask yourself the questions below to clarify your own needs:

    *   When did you become aware of a difference in sex drive?
    *   How much sex would you need to have?
    *   How much sex would you like to have?
    *   Are your sexual needs being met?

- What does sex mean to you?
- What do you think sex means to your partner? Is it just a physical act or more?
- Without blaming your partner, what do you think are some of the reasons there is a difference in sexual interest or desire?
- What will make you want to have sex more—is it the quality of sex, duration of foreplay, or frequency you would like to work on and perhaps adjust?
- Are your attitudes and beliefs about sex and sexuality supporting you?

3. **Rule out hormonal imbalance**

   While having a different level of desire doesn't necessarily mean something is wrong, it could mean that there is. When was the last time you had a thorough medical check-up? Once you rule out hormonal imbalance, you may wish to consider getting professional support by way of a clinical sexologist or sex therapist to better facilitate your inner dialogue or even the discussion process with your partner.

4. **Monitor your lifestyle patterns**

   Are you too stressed, tired and busy? There is some truth in eating healthily, getting moderate exercise and having sufficient rest. All these help regulate your hormones and affect your sexual desire.

5. Talk to your partner

The obvious is not always easy. You need to be able to communicate in a manner that is not blaming. It is about being committed to staying together and possibly taking baby steps towards where both of you agree would be towards the desired outcome.

Perhaps you could write a letter to your partner about how you are feeling and ask for a response in a similar fashion. Writing can help open up more possibilities. If talking about it is too much of a struggle or talking does not seem to help, you should seek out a counsellor or therapist.

6. Get creative

Have you always wondered why sex is lacking romance, emotional connection, all the sensory enhancement that you always long for such as music, essence oil, lingerie, etc? You are the other 50% in the relationship, and can make sex better by implementing some changes!

For instance, because a woman tends to take a longer time to be sexually aroused, you can get yourself into the mood by setting the scene for yourself—slow bath, candles, low lights. You may also wish to ask for a massage from your partner. On days that you are not in the mood for penetrative sex, you can offer to perform oral sex on him instead. You can research online and experiment different fellatio techniques on him. What this does is ensure that giving oral sex to him is fun and interesting for both of you. In no time, you will be better at giving oral sex and also learn more about what your partner likes.

Remember, being in a relationship where the sex drives are different is actually very common. With some considered talking, planning, and willingness to compromise, you can get past it. This could be a temporary problem, or it can be something that you struggle with for the entire duration of the relationship. Either way, remember that the love you have for each other will help you work through this problem. Sex matters!

Q *My wife is not interested in sex. What should I do?*

A It is normal for couples to have differences in their sexual desire. It is important for couples to begin by having a honest discussion about how often they need to have sex versus how often they would ideally like to have sex. There needs to be a conversation about the role sex plays in a relationship and why it is important. Stress, anxiety and tiredness are very real factors that affect the sex lives of Singaporeans. It's hard to get in the mood or have any real desire when you've been working long hours.

Women tend to blame their lower sexual desire for the lack of sexual activity in their lives. It is possible to bypass her lack of mental desire by physically stimulating and arousing her. Hence there is the possibility that when you incorporate more touch in your life, your female partner is more likely to get aroused and, consequently increase the possibility of having more sex in your life.

Q *What's with the typical "I have a headache" excuse to get out of going at it?*

A Rather than dismissing them as excuses, how about acknowledging them as a genuine health issue especially if they are happening frequently? Expressing your concern for your partner and coming up with ways to work through the problems will be more productive than becoming resentful over them. Your partner may wish to consult a physician to rule out any possibility that this is indeed something more serious. You may also wish to let your partner know that sex can actually help with headaches. Sex encourages your body to release endorphins, having a similar effect on your body as morphine. Also orgasms help improve blood flow which may alleviate the symptoms.

Q *Does oral contraception cause a drop in libido?*

A Because of its convenience, the female oral contraception, more famously just known as "the pill", remains the most popular method of birth control in the United States. It contains various hormones to suppress ovulation by suppressing the release of the hormones by the pituitary gland. They can cause changes in the libido of a woman as well as mood swings and weight gain. However health benefits of the pill include lowered risk of ovarian cancer, endometrial cancer, acne and pelvic inflammatory disease. For the vast majority of women, the health risks from unintended pregnancies far outweigh any risk from the pill.

Sexual Addictions

1. **How do you differentiate between what my mum used to call "oversexed" and sexual addiction?**

   The definitive DSM-IV-TR, which is the latest version of the Diagnostic and Statistical Manual of Mental Disorders published by the American Psychiatric Association, does not recognise sexual addiction as a diagnosis. Conventional wisdom among therapists has long been that there is no such thing as a sex addict. I would prefer to refer to what is commonly called sexual addiction as a form of obsessive compulsive disorder and refer to it as sexual compulsivity, as a more accurate term.

   The difference between somebody who is sexually compulsive and "oversexed" is that the former cannot stop his behaviour, whilst the latter might have a higher sexual drive than "normal" people. I question "normal" because all human beings are born sexual and there is no limit placed on the frequency of sexual encounters humans can engage in. Just as there is no limit to a human being's freedom of sexual expression. Also just because somebody has a higher sex drive, or libido, than others doesn't necessarily mean he or she is engaged in any self harming behaviour and ought to be stopped.

2. What are the signs of sexual addiction?

Sexual behaviour becomes a problem when it is repeated often enough to interfere with normal daily living and functionality. This might include adverse interferences with relationships, work, friendships and lifestyle.

Tell-tale signs are when the individual is spending long periods of time over sex-related activities; feels unable to control the sexual behaviour or reduce its incidence; and is distressed and depressed about it.

3. How much of sexual addiction is about power? How much about emotional need?

What other experts refer to as a "sex addict" may actually be a manifestation of narcissism. A narcissist attempts to prove his sexual superiority by engaging in a pattern of repeated sexual relationships with women with no emotional attachment.

Narcissists lack empathy for others and possess an exaggerated sense of entitlement, self-importance or self worth including engaging in repeated sexual encounters to exert control over others. Narcissists are addicted to power, attention and fear — not sex.

People with sexual compulsive behaviour often use sex as an escape from other problems such as anxiety, stress, depression and social isolation. And certainly this is to fill a physical and emotional gap not met elsewhere.

4. **Can women be sexual addicts? And is the stigma
    worse for them? Emotional and material costs also
    worse?**

    Yes women can be sexual compulsives, though it is
    most commonly men. Physiologically women tend
    to have a lower sex drive, and there is nothing wrong
    with having a high sex drive. However because society
    in general tends to expect women to suppress, not
    express their sexuality, the chances of stigmatisation is
    definitely there. Why is it that men who sleep around a
    lot are "studs" and women who do the same are "sluts"?
    It has a lot to do with cultural programming and
    societal stereotyping.

5. **What is the treatment for sex addiction? Unlike
    alcohol, I don't think it's something someone can
    just give up altogether.**

    Treatment may depend on the cause. Behavioural
    treatments have been found to be helpful. Interventions
    like the 12-step programme which can be effective for
    some compulsivities has not always worked for sexually
    compulsive clients. A doctor may be able to treat
    depressional aspects of sexual addiction with medication.

Sex Without Orgasm—What's the Point?

If you mention the words "sex without orgasm" to a man, it's most likely you would get a blank stare or an honest retort thrown back at you: "What is the point?". Indeed, there seems to always be a purpose, target, objective or end goal in everything that a man does—even when it comes to sex. You may attribute it to social conditioning, cultural expectations imposed upon him, or even the neurological wiring of his brain by testosterone.

For a man, sex without orgasm may seem pointless. The fact is sex feels good, orgasms make sex better, and sex without orgasm can feel incomplete—perhaps akin to champagne without the bubbles, a wedding without the cake, or even a ten-course dinner without the dessert. Yet, for others, the orgasm might be an unattainable goal.

How would you like it if the roles were reversed?

If you are a man who cannot imagine sex without being able to attain orgasm, get this: majority of women (70% according to most studies) cannot reach orgasm through vaginal intercourse alone.

Since most of the vagina's sensory nerve endings are located in its first couple of inches, penetration may not be enough to bring her over "the edge" to ecstasy. The vagina is much more responsive to targeted stimulation. So, if you are a woman who cannot achieve orgasm through penile-vaginal penetration, why would you want to have (simply goal-oriented) sex?

Many women enjoy vaginal intercourse because of the nice feeling of fullness, the emotional closeness, and from the intimacy from pleasing one's partner. Satisfaction is in the eyes of the beholder. A large percentage of women whom have never had orgasms are still able to describe their sex lives as very satisfying.

Do you think you can lighten up on the quest for the orgasm?

Sex is not just about reproduction, or about setting a quota to maintain marital obligations or harmony in a relationship. "Real sex" should be about what is stimulating, exciting and satisfying for both persons, whether that is achieved through intercourse or by other means. Setting a goal to have intercourse for the sole reason to reach orgasm is not only an unrealistic goal but is also going to keep you from having sex you really can enjoy.

The techniques that work in helping you reach orgasm can change on a yearly, monthly, even daily basis—depending on what is going on in your body and life. What works can be individual, and may also vary from partner to partner. There is no one activity that guarantees anyone will reach orgasm either. Being concerned about what is "supposed" to work or is "normal" is a good way to prevent yourself and your partner from just appreciating the experience.

What's love got to do with it?

What does and does not "work" for you sexually is not just about the sexual chemistry, physical techniques or emotional connection. Is it possible to love deeply, but not feel "fireworks" sexually? The dynamics *during* sex matters— for instance, is your partner emotionally distant when you want closeness, too gentle when you desire something more aggressive, or the reverse?

Many people assume that the stars will cosmically align, and amazing sex—including multitudes of orgasms—will happen as long as there is love. They assume that sex is a wholly instinctive act, when in reality it is learned behaviour, and is one of those activities that tends to take time and practice to get really awesome. Therefore, take the time to experiment and explore each other, learn to communicate about sex and respond accordingly.

What are the other factors causing a lack of orgasm?

It takes time to get to know your body, just as it takes time to learn about a partner's body. Older people are actually able to have orgasms of the same quality or with the same frequency often because they are more comfortable with their bodies, so they are able to relax into the idea of having sex, willing to go with what feels good, and care less about what they "should" be doing.

Once again, focusing on what feels good and is pleasurable, even if and when it doesn't result in orgasm, is important. Stressing too much about coming could just be what is causing us not to have an orgasm. It is also not easy to have an orgasm if you are uptight, tired, stressed or unhappy in your relationship.

Having said all this, having an orgasm is a lovely feeling. The build-up, release and resulting feelings of bliss (and the cuddling that can help sustain a natural high) are absolutely wonderful. You are entitled to it. If you are concerned that something physical might be interfering with your ability to have an orgasm, you should consult your health care professional.

May you enjoy the sex you have—with or without an orgasm.

How to help her attain orgasm

- Setting the stage—the lighting, candles, music—all help turn women on.
- Give her oral sex—because it feels good!
- Take your time. Remember the importance of foreplay—many women need more than 20 minutes of foreplay to reach their sexual peak.
- Incorporate intercourse with something else—such as manual clitoral stimulation, using of a vibrator or her touching herself.
- The woman-on-top position allows her to be in charge of the angle of penetration, and can provide more direct clitoral stimulation resulting in orgasms being more likely.
- Reassure her that she is beautiful, wonderful, and turns you on.
- Encourage your partner to show you how to do what works for her, and vice versa!

Straying
Your tail is showing

What causes men to stray, and what women should know

Cheating in a relationship is otherwise known as "straying" and "infidelity", or if one is married, "adultery" or having an "extra martial affair". The third wheel in the relationship is usually referred to as the "girlfriend", "lover" or "mistress". What makes a man stray? Is there something that can be done? What should women know about cheating?

The simple answer of why men stray is this: he wants to. Also he can and knows he can get away with it. He travels internationally for work, is expected to socialise with clients, needs to be contactable, and has the latest technological gadgets at his fingertips. There are opportunities aplenty for him to meet, keep in touch with and romance other women.

The usual suspected reasons might vary from the man experiencing a midlife crisis; getting sexually bored; desiring the excitement of an affair; wishing to keep the status quo of a current relationship; to not being fully committed to the relationship or testing "waters" before ending a relationship. Additionally, these are three areas women should be watching out for:

1. **Lifestyle changes**

    Things seldom remain the same especially in long-term relationships. Shifts in lifestyle can create an upheaval be it a new position that requires long hours with added responsibilities, or moving to a new home in a new city. It could be an unforeseen financial disaster, the birth of a child, or death of a family member. In addition, you no longer look and behave the same as during your courtship days.

Adjustments have to be made in tandem with drastic life changes. This is the period, more than ever, where there should be ongoing communication of fears and concerns. Change should be dealt with together so that the relationship is actually strengthened. When you neglect to support your partner during stressful periods of his life, or worse start leading entirely separate lives, it weakens a relationship.

2. Lack of sexual intimacy

Sex is an integral part of a relationship. Should you reduce or stop having sex, and intimacy is not nurtured, the relationship will wither and die over time. Admittedly it can be challenging to find the time for sex if both of you are busy juggling work, family and household, yet it is important to give intimacy a priority. Put sex into your schedule and prepare yourself for it as you would a date. By being more prepared, both of you can be assured of a better experience.

When sex is explosive and mind-blowing, it cements you to your partner in a very powerful way, and thus opens the door for more intimacy. Hence intimacy and great sex feed each other. Maintaining sexual excitement takes planning and effort. Text your partner, and tell him how eager you are to be with him tonight. Leave naughty notes for each other. Wear lingerie, not just for him, but for you too! Consider sex coaching from a compassionate trained sexologist.

3. Lack of emotional intimacy

Emotional intimacy is about the ability to share one's fears, dreams and pains. Sharing makes one vulnerable and can feel extremely risky and scary. Most people don't like that and intentionally avoid being vulnerable— perhaps by keeping themselves busy with their career— and thereby run away from intimacy.

However it is vital to keep trying—being conscious of the words you are using and what they mean. Share about each other's day including your thoughts and feelings. Unless there is consistent dialogue, you can grow apart with time, even turning into strangers. Also once the intellectual and emotional sharing in the relationship stops, intimacy and passion in sex will end soon after.

If it happens… it's a chance for change

Many women react blindly when they first find out about the affair. They go through the stages of denial, outrage and disappointment before finally acknowledging the reality of betrayal. My advice is not to do anything until you have a frank discussion, reassess and take a broader view before you decide to stay or leave. One of the ironies about an affair is that it creates an opportunity to have some honest conversations about what works and hasn't worked in the relationship for some time.

For some women, staying is the right decision. For others, what feels right may be to leave. Each woman must make her own choice. He must be on board for a relationship to heal. And you should never have to feel you need to explain or defend your decision to anyone (other than your children) as to why you chose to leave or to stay with a man who cheats.

***

The monogamous model for relationship has not existed through all societies and time. More so in our Asian culture, we are exposed to concepts like polygamy where Muslim men can have up to four wives; and *patriarchal* systems where the father or eldest male is head of the household, having authority over women and children and expected to continue the male line or family name. Affluent men of modern times have second wives or mistresses and explain it with reasons such as desire to take care/protect the woman, loneliness, need for variety, desire to continue the family name and so on.

A saying I have heard goes like this: "Even if I love Chicken Rice, I will still get tired of eating Chicken Rice everyday." Whichever way you look at it, much of the rationale for straying is centred on the man—and his sexual pleasure and desires—not the woman's.

Culturally in Asia, straying appears more acceptable because of how common it is.

According to San Francisco psychotherapist, Jack Morin from his book *The Erotic Mind**, he developed an "erotic equation" where: Attraction (A) plus obstacles (O) leads to excitement (E). Straying or having an extra martial affair is certainly exciting because of the obstacles including the risks of being found out—real or perceived.

$$A + O = E$$

Morin also suggested that sexual obstacles in one's youth create lifelong scripts for arousal, while a range of feelings including exuberance, anxiety and anger can intensify arousal. Meaning what is arousing for one in his younger days may become an erotic theme that runs through one's life e.g. a shoe fetish.

Understanding our peak sexual experiences and fantasies offers the greatest opportunity for self-discovery and the possibility of revitalising sexual experiences. Morin advises readers to confront the unresolved feelings that produce "troublesome turn-ons" and offers a seven-step guide to modifying or expanding one's erotic patterns.

* Morin, J. (1997) *The Erotic Mind: Unlock the Inner Sources of Sexual Passion and Fulfillment*, HarperCollins Publishers, Inc, New York USA, pp. 341.

Morin observed that passion is hardly guaranteed in long-term relationships; but instead advises couples to recognise and address the interactive tension between intimacy and sexual desire.

Q *Is it alright to have sex with my ex-girlfriend's best friend even though she says she's "cool with it"?*

A Are you talking about sex or pursing a romantic and sexual relationship with this new person? In deciding, you may wish to consider how long ago and for how long the dating took place, the reason for the break-up and whether this new person is worth losing your friendship over. Has your ex truly moved on—is she happily in love? Timing counts. Lastly, did your ex share intimate details of your relationship with her? Do you want to go there? At the end of the day, you have to decide based on what you think is best for you.

Vaginismus
When a woman's body says: "No entry"

When I began my practice, a girlfriend admitted that until she heard it from the horse's mouth (i.e. me), she had always thought that vaginismus was a myth—a disease that was made up, or had been eradicated in the 1980s, and most definitely did not exist in modern day.

In fact, vaginismus is a very real sexual concern that women experience, and more common than we might think.

Vaginismus is the instantaneous tightening of the muscles around the vagina when penetration of the vagina is attempted, making penetration difficult, painful or impossible. This involuntary reaction happens because the body perceives penetration as upsetting, painful (in anticipation of it), frightening or dangerous. The mind may be willing, but the body is screaming "No entry!"

Both the woman with vaginismus and her partner can feel very distressed, helpless, frustrated and inadequate. She might experience self-blame and a loss of self-confidence for her inability to have penetrative sex. Inaccurate sexual information and the lack of understanding of the woman's body will worsen the condition, often leading to alienation and even break-ups.

When Cindy*, 28, came to see me, she had already sought treatment from several gynaecologists who had examined her, found nothing physically wrong with her and told her to "Just relax". One doctor suggested she use a dilator kit, which helps expand the vaginal passage gradually, but Cindy rejected it as being too intimidating.

Melissa*, 35 and married for 10 years, has the same condition. She came to see me frustrated with the lack of concrete results having paid top dollar to see the best gynaecologists. Melissa was examined each visit and instructed to do Kegel exercises (which consists of contracting and relaxing the muscles that form part of the pelvic floor)—but not told why. Like Cindy, there was little dialogue between doctor and patient.

Realising that the cause was psychological, I made sure both ladies understood their sexual anatomy (what is what and where), and the sexual response cycle (what happens during sex). We began a conversation about what she can expect to feel and what can be done to alleviate pain during penetrative sex; this conversation continued through the course of our sessions. The process to demystify what sex was and deal directly with their condition had begun.

I taught my clients a combination of breathing and relaxation techniques, physical callisthenics and pelvic exercises which they were to do each day. The purpose was to retrain them to develop awareness and comfort with their bodies as well as to sensitise and strengthen their pelvic muscles. I encouraged Cindy and Melissa to each keep a journal so they could monitor their own progress, record any feelings and memories that came up, and to better remember what they would like to share with me during our sessions.

By our second session, Cindy said she felt "different" physically but was unable to articulate how exactly. In her determination to overcome vaginismus, she had already been practising vaginal insertion with her dildo. I encouraged her to continue her daily practice. Also, I suggested that rather than push or force an object into her vagina, she could simply hold the dildo at the entrance of her vagina, incorporating her breathing and relaxation exercises, so her vagina would "open up" and "receive" naturally.

Similarly, I encouraged Melissa to purchase a dildo, smaller than the vibrator she already had, and to practise at home. She was to attempt penetration after having achieved her orgasm through self stimulation. When Melissa emailed to say she was able to do self penetration with her dildo without pain, I knew she was close to a breakthrough.

In our third session, Cindy wondered aloud how penetrative sex would change her and her relationship. I was secretly delighted how our conversation had progressed from what sex was about, and dealing with pain, to what might change for her emotionally when penetrative sex did happen.

Cindy was unable to see me for a few weeks due to work. However, when I next heard from her, it was fantastic news! She had been successful in penetrative sex with her partner for the first time.

Melissa had amazing news of her own! She was able to have successful penetrative sex with her husband before our third session—thrice in fact, each time better than the previous encounter. She was overjoyed: "I cannot thank you enough.

You are truly God-sent. I have been struggling for so long. This is better than winning the one-million-dollar lottery."

In her thank you note, Cindy wrote, "If I had not met you, I am certain that I would still be in the same position I was a few months ago, struggling with something that I thought was near impossible."

I saw Cindy for a fourth time where we discussed methods to better enjoy the sex she was already having. At our third session, Melissa was radiant, glowing with joy and more beautiful than I have seen her. Her husband and her are communicating more, happier than ever and enjoying every sexual experience. Both ladies are well on their way to greater sexual pleasure and satisfaction, and embracing life as a complete being.

Miracle worker, I am not. I provided Cindy and Melissa with the education, encouragement and individualised treatment based on techniques that have been proven to work. Vaginismus is actually highly treatable.

Names have been changed to maintain client confidentiality. Explicit permission was received to tell their story so as to benefit and help more women.

201: BETTER SEX

Conscious Connecting

How about going within yourselves and reconnecting with each other consciously? How would you like to rekindle your romance through authentic touch?

There are four essential types of touching:

1. **Giving**

   In this touch, you are essentially delivering the kind of touch which your partner likes based on their explicit request—to the right part of the body and how it should be done; including the grip and strength. This may be a back rub, shoulder massage or body cradle. The giver's intention is to be generous and to nurture the recipient. Givers can solicit feedback from the receiver, so they can improve their techniques.

2. **Receiving**

   Conversely the other person is being given touch and actively receiving touch. The receiver's role is to be open to experiencing pleasure through being touched. Expressions of pleasure, such as smiling and making noises as well as gratitude to the giver, will reinforce that the touch is desirable and wanted. It is important that the receiver learns to understand their own body's responses. Receivers may give feedback to the giver so the touch can be even better next time.

3. **Absorbing**

   With this touch, the absorber is the one doing the touching, while the one being touched is the allower. The absorber is focused on what he or she can feel through touching, rather than giving what the allower wants. There is still authentic consent while the absorber is activating the muscles of their body through, for instance, the use of the back of the arm, wrist, hand, palm and fingertips. The absorber's role is to enjoy the range of pleasure possible through the physical connection.

4. **Allowing**

   The person being touched is allowing him or herself to be touched by the absorber without judgement or evaluation. In surrendering, the allower can effectively "melt" into taking the touch right into his or her body, and essentially be able to attain an even deeper state of relaxation. This surrender may take place not just physically but also mentally.

Benefits of conscious touching

- **To ask:** We become fixed in giving the type of touch which we think our partner likes, wants or had asked for before. We forget that needs, wants and desires can change. Sometimes, we ourselves get caught up with what we are used to—and forget to ask.

- **To receive:** One partner is usually more comfortable giving than receiving. Through deliberate practice, it is possible to become more comfortable with receiving and asking for what is a more pleasurable touch.

- **To explore:** Absorbing reminds us that it is also important to give the touch we like and to experience pleasure through the touches we enjoy giving our partners. In practising absorbing touching, we are nudged into remembering the joy of an exploratory touch.

- **To come alive:** Absorbing and allowing touches allow us to feel more sensation in our bodies. When we feel more, and when we can also feel the pleasure of touching our partner, this is when the "magic" happens.

Practising these four different types of touches will clarify how you relate with your partner. Conscious connecting will bring a new level of presence and sensuality to all your touches together. Go reach out and touch—today.

Q *Sometimes women just want to cuddle but are not in the mood for sex. Why is it so hard for men to understand that not every hug and kiss leads to sex?*

A He does understand but he cannot help the physiological reaction that his body has from being touched or being around you. Just because he has an erection with you does not mean that he has to have sex there and then. If in doubt, ask. You might well be surprised that even though he is having an erection, he does not necessarily want sex.

Q *Why is the power of touch so important in a relationship? Even on a day-to-day basis, how does "touch" keep a couple feeling connected, so that it carries through to their sexual relationship?*

A To better understand the power of touch, one can benefit from reading the popular book *The Five Languages of Love* by Gary Chapman of which one of the love languages identified is physical touch. Individuals who have physical touch as their primary love language actually "feel" love and feel nurtured in a relationship most when touched. Even for those who are not used to touch, it is well established that touch has great health and healing benefits. It can lower stress levels, lessen anxiety, and help a myriad of other physical disorders.

One cannot have sex without touch so touch actually keeps the physical connection between two strong as well as stimulates the continued growth of loving relationships. It is the conduit between two individuals that allows them to connect as one. If you desire more touch in your relationship, acknowledge that you feel less connected and want a way to spend more time touching your partner, and help them feel loved.

Q *Why is kissing important?*

A Lips are proven to be 200 times more sensitive than even the finGers, with more nerve endings per unit area of skin. Hence it is not surprising that kissing of the lips can lead to an orgasm.

Kissing releases endorphins and neurotransmitters (chemicals) like Dopamine, responsible for emotional arousal and Noradrenaline for physical arousal. Besides triggering an emotional response, kissing is fun (an erotic experience), natural (usually a prelude to intercourse), playful (introducing the bodies to intimacy) and progressive (builds anticipation and excitement). Kissing is also the first sexual activity to diminish when couples are growing apart.

Kissing trivia:

Kissing

- Enables your jaw to open wider;
- Strengthens your jaw;
- Builds muscles in the tongue;
- Requires 20 muscles working in co-ordination;
- Hickeys are broken blood vessels that rise to the surface of the skin after someone has sucked on it for about 30 seconds.

Tips to make kissing more exciting

- Place an ice cube inside your mouth and gently slide it into your lover's mouth while kissing.
- Put your all into everything you do with a full body kiss.
- Be gentle and tease your lover by moving your tongue and lips gently up and down, around the front and the back of the neck.

- Always have fresh smelling breath.
- Get a sense of whether or not the person is interested in sharing a kiss.
- Plan ahead of time where you will place your head and lips.

Kissing no-no's?

- Don't slobber. The amount of moisture should remain the same as your normal state.
- Don't tense up your lips. Allow your lips to relax, not sloppy, but loose.
- Don't squash your lover's lips. It hurts and makes it difficult for them to respond.
- Regardless of how they are responding to you, go in for a kiss and lay one on them.

Getting Feedback after Sex

Because we are not psychics

Sex is not a one-way experience. I would like to suggest ways in which we can get feedback from our partner after a sexual experience. And when I say sexual experience, I am not limiting it to just penetrative sex.

Open-ended questions

You can begin by asking your partner what the sexual experience was like:

"Sweetheart, how was it for you?" or *"How was it just now?"*
If feedback is restricted to one-word answers or not forthcoming, you can elaborate by saying:

"Ok… You know, I would really like to hear what you like about it and what would make it better. Could you share more with me?"

An open-ended question allows for your partner to communicate as little or as much as desired. Breaking the questions down might be easier:

"How was it?"
"What was good about it?"
"What would make it better?"

Remember if you ask, be emotionally and mentally prepared for the answer—whatever it may be. If you appear defensive or react negatively, you are effectively being counterproductive and shutting out your partner at a critical time.

All of us will do well to bear this in mind: Don't take it personally. There is no right or wrong answer. We are different physically on a day-to-day basis—depending on our fitness level, what is going on in our lives, and how it affects our mood. What doesn't feel right or good on one day could well feel quite different on another day. The feedback you receive is not a judgement of your character or sexual prowess. There is always room for improvement and a large part of it comes from understanding your partner, from their likes and dislikes; turn on and offs; as well as needs, wants and desires—and it probably has very little to do with you.

Don't be too hard on yourself. Constant, open and authentic communication will bring you closer.

Closed-ended questions

All of us would have inadvertently said something to hurt someone. Hence, when you try to get sexual feedback from your partner, their own fears of hurting you will come into play. They are not just worried of potentially hurting you, but also have a disbelief that you are genuinely willing and open to hear from them. It will take a while before your partner will begin to talk more openly about his or her sexual experiences.

If you have limited success with open-ended questions, don't give up. This is where you move onto closed-ended questions such as:

"Did you notice when I did…..?" (Yes or No)

"Did you like it when I did it?" (If your partner does not

remember, you could imitate what you did previously.)
"Was your orgasm the same, less or more intense than the
last time?" (There is only one answer.)
This is where you can encourage further dialogue by
reverting to a few open-ended questions:
"That's interesting. Could you tell me more?"
"Really? Why (gently) do you think that is so?"

If your partner asks you why you have recently begun asking
so many questions after sex, you could reply:

> *"I really want to learn more about you, what works and*
> *what would make it better… and I think one of the ways to*
> *do so is by talking about it. I really want to know because I*
> *care about you."*

Or:

> *"I want us to be able to talk about sex and our sexual*
> *experiences. This is one way we can learn more about each*
> *other. Is it okay?"*

This is not an interrogation. There is no point pushing it if
your partner is clearly uncomfortable talking about sex. Try
again the next time, and the next. What you want to do is
begin to open more dialogue about sex, and stopping that
dialogue when your partner wishes to do so is a part of it.
You will notice that with each attempt to discuss your sexual
experiences, it will become easier. It takes time and it is well
worth it to go slow.

Scale of 1 to 10

If your partner is not forthcoming when you use open-ended questions to get sexual feedback, or if you wish to get clearer answers, you can try using a scale. This is how you might begin:

> "On a scale of one to ten, ten being the highest, what do you think of this (technique/position/etc.)? Give it a number."
> "How would you rank today's (experience/orgasm, etc) compared to the last time?"

> Example: "Oh, I am just curious, why is this an eight, and that a six? What is it about this that makes it an eight? There is no right or wrong answer, baby (or add your own pet name). I love you and I want to learn more about what you like."

Using the scale method, you can drill down to get more specific feedback. You can use the scale to ask your partner, "How horny are you?" or "How much would you like to have sex today?" to get a sense of their desire for sex at that particular time. If you are at a level of ten and your partner a four, agree on a sexual activity that both of you would be willing to experience.

Or ask "How tired are you on a scale of one to ten, ten being the highest?", to better understand how your partner is feeling physically, the amount of emotional support expected of you that evening, as well as whether sex is a possibility.

Code words

Couples who have been together for some time say that they can gauge the "mood" or even the response of their partner—most of the time. This is not foolproof. Unless you are a psychic or mindreader, communication is indeed the key to a better sexual life.

How would you like to be able to communicate clearly, accurately, every single time on matters important to you? Consider using code words. A code word is a word or a phrase designed to convey a predetermined meaning to a receptive audience, while remaining inconspicuous to the uninitiated.

Take for instance: "Red", "Yellow" and "Green".

No prizes for guessing that "Green" means "Yes", "Go ahead", or "It's okay". "Yellow" could represent "Slow down", "You are in a danger zone", or "Back up a bit"; whilst "Red" is for "Stop right now", "Danger", or "No go".

You can use code words to indicate arousal (getting there), plateau (don't stop), or orgasm (release). They can state your level of readiness for penetrative sex or indicate a state of distress, such as if an anxiety or panic attack is about to happen.

You will do well to overcome any resistance in coming up with code words and using them if you explain that the use of code words does not mean you are not in love or distrust your partner, but simply a better way to communicate where you are. Code words help take the display of emotion out of your words.

Open- or closed-ended questions are simple enough to use. Incorporating a scale and code words to give or receive feedback might seem silly to you, yet they do work. Your partner needs to believe that you are receptive to sexual feedback. Encouraging your partner to open up and express sexual feelings and thoughts takes time. The more you communicate, the more you learn and understand about what makes your partner tick. Consequently, this increases your chances of having many wonderful sexual experiences. Keep at it. Good luck.

3 tips on how a man can caress a woman's breasts and nipples to stimulate her

- She will only welcome focused touch when sufficiently aroused. Don't always go straight for the nipples.
- Try to avoid anything that resembles a breast examination. The side of her boobs are areas full of nerve endings that are often under-touched.
- Just like when you finger a woman, you want to warm the stove before you put anything in. Mix things up from soft stroking, squeezing (but not like an overeager teenager), licking, sucking (but not like an infant) and perhaps a nipple tweak.

5 tips to approaching her breast

- Warm her up. Fondle or massage her breasts.
- Kiss. Make sure these are gentle lip kisses to her nipples.
- Lick. Apply short, wet and frantic licks on her erect nipple or around.

- Suck on her breasts. Kiss her nipple and then slowly lower your mouth until you have a mouthful.
- Bite. You might be surprised that applying a bit of teeth against her breast when she is sufficiently aroused will feel nice. Do so gently first and apply more pressure if she responds favourably.

3 tips on how a man can caress a woman's butt to stimulate her

- Get your partner to lie face down, whether clothed or not. You can begin by slowly kneading the muscles of the back and neck—the farthest place away from her butt—before moving south.
- After a few minutes, begin to move tantalisingly close to the top of the cheeks and occasionally reach down to stroke deep onto each cheek. You may tease around the anus—keep it light, move down to the legs and quickly move to the feet.
- Even if you do not penetrate the anus, pouring or squeezing lubricant between the anus connection allows for a different sensation. This is a very sensitive area and your partner is likely to give a strong signal as to how you should proceed next. Lightly stroke the entire area. You may wish to tease the genital area as well. This dual stimulation is likely to elicit another strong response.

Q *Can a woman feel when a man cums inside herself?*

A It's common for women not to feel it when their partner ejaculates inside of them. This is because most of nerve endings are close to the vaginal entrance rather than deeper inside. However there are many women who can tell when their partner is ejaculating such as from the tension in the body, facial expression, sound or other ways.

Q *Is it hygienic to have sex during her period?*

A Menstrual blood is an entirely natural bodily fluid and does not affect a man's penis or a woman's reproductive tract. During her period, a woman's cervix opens to allow blood to pass through creating the perfect pathway for bacteria to travel deep inside the pelvic cavity. The vagina's pH during menstruation is less acidic. Hence there are increased risks of passing and receiving sexually transmitted diseases and infections during this time. There is also a chance of pregnancy. But this does not mean it is unhygienic. It is entirely alright to have sex during a woman's period as long as you are engaging in safe and protected sexual intercourse.

Q *My wife and I keep sex quiet because of the kids, but I can't climax. What should I do?*

A Besides waiting for the kids to be asleep or putting on music to mask the sounds of pleasure you are making, how about having a baby-sitter and scheduling date nights with your wife? Scheduling sex allows both of you to be in a better frame of mind for a positive experience. You could either stay home when the kids are being taken care of, or choose to whisk her to a boutique or budget hotel of your choice. The time and effort spent towards preparing for the date will be well worth the peace of mind you will have.

Q *Do I still need to use a condom if she is on birth control pills?*

A The Pill is an effective method of birth control when used properly. However it does not protect against HIV or other sexually transmitted infections, which the condom can. Some women are prone to yeast and vaginal infections and condoms can ease related anxieties, helping to make sex even better. Even couples in monogamous relationships I know of continue using condoms because of the convenience in cleaning up afterwards. There are so many types of condoms on the market—size, textured and flavoured—which are just as safe as the plain ones. I am certain you will be able to find a right one.

Q *How can i tell if she's faking an orgasm?*

A An orgasm is not just a physical experience, it happens in your body, mind, possibly even spirit. And there is no single definition of orgasm. Some tell-tale signs of an orgasmic response might include increased heart rate and blood pressure, increased muscle tension, a flush of her skin, as well as a release of tension followed sometimes by a feeling of deep relaxation. On the other hand, she might experience one or several of these things and not "feel" she had an orgasm. Trying to figure out if she had an orgasm can also be a dead end. If she had one, does that mean you stop exploring other ways of getting her to feel good or have orgasms?

Q *Do women prefer to orgasm simultaneously with their guys?*
A Women tend to need more foreplay in order to attain an orgasm. To attain a simultaneous orgasm, she might need to learn how to speed up her arousal, and for you to slow down your sexual response. A gauge is anywhere between 15 to 30 minutes of arousal for her. Simultaneous orgasm is actually incredibly difficult to time, and is usually the exception than the norm.

Q *How can you get your sex lives in synch e.g. he wakes up in the morning with an erection, but she prefers sex at night? At night, he's often too tired! And in the mornings, she's too busy!*
A Men usually like morning sex because after a good night's sleep, their body is relaxed and the blood flow to the penis allows it to be erect more easily. The hardness of his penis also gives him greater sexual confidence.

Communicate to really understand each other's body clock preference. It is not good enough to think you know why your partner prefers sex at a different time of the day. Pretend you are a detective and ask "why" questions until you begin to see things from his point of view. Once you understand, the "pain" of having morning or evening sex is diminished.

For ladies, it would be unrealistic for me to suggest that you force yourself to become an energiser bunny in the mornings. Find a half way point where

- On days he is too tired to have sex in the evenings, you wake up early on agreed days of the week (say you agree the evening before to have morning sex).
- Or he has forewarning (say as he goes about the day) that you would like to have sex that evening. Both of you can begin preparing mentally for sex that evening and look forward to that encounter.
- If sex is just not happening despite the above efforts, consider scheduling sex so both parties can have more time to prepare for sex. For instance, the man might wish to have a quick nap during lunchtime so he has more energy in the evening. Or she goes to bed early for their morning quickie. It is about compromises i.e. taking turns (this week we have morning sex, next time, we have it in the evening).

For all you know, you might be so pleased with his satisfied smile and the positive effects morning sex has to your relationship that waking up earlier for sex becomes a non-issue but you won't know unless you try it, with a different attitude towards it.

Q *I often feel like peeing during sex. Is it okay to hold it in?*

A I usually get asked this only by women as during penetrative sex, her urethra is being stimulated, resulting in this peeing sensation. When a man is about to ejaculate, the opening to his bladder closes to prevent urine from mixing with semen. Men cannot urinate and ejaculate at the same time. Relax and go with the flow.

Q *My wife says my semen irritates her vagina. Is it my diet?*

A Semen allergy is a rare condition often misdiagnosed as a common yeast or herpes infection. The allergy usually causes pain, redness, burning and swelling of the outer vaginal area. Some women can also have hives all over the body, vomiting, diarrhoea, wheezing and difficulty with breathing. If she has existing allergies, there is a remote possibility that tiny particles of the food you ate earlier has made its way into your semen and are now irritating her vagina. However it is more likely that it has to do with the protein in your semen. Once accurately diagnosed by medical doctors, couples can be treated successfully.

Q *Does the woman-on-top position really make for better sex?*

A When the woman is on top, the man can relax, focus on his sensations, and surrender to his orgasmic pleasure. It also means he might not be able to last as long as the woman is dictating the pace and depth of thrusting. She will also have easier access to her clitoris if she desires added stimulation. Although this implies she should climax more readily, many women are not comfortable with this position. She might feel vulnerable, uncomfortable with being in the spotlight or awkward due to lack of sexual experience. Encourage her as with practice, this position will feel more natural. The missionary position (man-on-top) should be more comfortable for her.

Q *I am a virgin, and am getting married soon. Having no experience in sex, what are the fail-safe things I can do to "wow" her in bed?*

A Get over "wowing" her in bed—right now. The sex we have in our heads is almost always going to be nicer than reality. First time sex is rarely what we imagine it is to. Those who set high expectations for or of themselves will usually end up disappointed. I would rather that you focus on what is good touch for both of you—pleasure, never pain. Learn about sexual anatomy and prepare yourself mentally, physically and emotionally for sex in the meantime. Also go online and research "first time intercourse".

Q *I've been faking an orgasm but feel terrible about it. What can I do?*

A Many women don't orgasm every time and only a few can by intercourse alone. When you fake an orgasm, you are essentially putting on a show for the benefit of your partner. Your reasons could vary from "getting it over with", "sparing his feelings", misleading yourself with "what he doesn't know won't hurt", to the inner satisfaction of "pulling it off" and "getting away with it". Whatever your reasons, it is important to call a spade a space: you are lying to your partner, and more importantly to yourself.

Q *I'm tired of being only able to orgasm with clitoral stimulation. How can my husband make me orgasm with his penis?*

A During intercourse, it is the outer third of the vagina that is most stimulated. Some women are able to orgasm through this vaginal penetration. That is, vaginal orgasm — without clitoral stimulation.

However research has shown that (Shere Hite's 1976 survey of 3,000 women) only 30% of women can achieve orgasm through intercourse. The clitoris, with 8,000 nerve endings, is more sensitive than the vagina. For a woman's orgasm, her body's response is the same whether or not stimulation originates from the clitoris or the vagina. As such a clitoral orgasm rather than a vaginal orgasm is more likely.

In the large majority of women the position for intercourse and the way in which the clitoris is being stimulated through intercourse is not conducive to orgasm and there is no way that intercourse alone can produce an orgasm. As such rather than being fixated on penile vaginal orgasm, acknowledge that there are different types of orgasms. Take the pressure off yourself, relax and enjoy the sensations. The important thing is that you should be having orgasms whenever you want them—and that you should be enjoying them hugely.

Q *Do aphrodisiac foods really work?*

A Aphrodisiacs are substances that supposedly enhance erotic perceptions and sexual performance. In virtually all societies, people have sought such agents and have attributed magical or powerful properties to unusual substances, like ground rhinoceros horn. It is controversial whether any single substance has singular and specific effects in enhancing sexual arousal and orgasm. Whether the effect is real, minimal or non-existent may well be a self-fulfilling prophecy. An agent that effectively stimulates sexual interest and response is not the same as an agent that non-specifically lessens inhibitions. An example is alcohol which is probably the most available mind-altering agent and is often reported to lessen inhibitions and enhance sexual feelings. The assumption is that alcohol is relatively safe yet it affects people in different ways, with individuals having different tolerances. So far there is no herb or witch's potion has been proven to be a true aphrodisiac. Don't take my word for it—experiment for yourself and let me know how it goes for you!

Q *I've always loved vaginal sex, but my husband is not very well endowed, so I've had to rely on clitoral stimulation alone.*

A Some 80% of women can only orgasm through clitoral stimulation and it has nothing to do with whether your husband is well endowed at all. There are some sexual positions such as woman-on-top which can help you to achieve orgasm better as you are in charge of the speed as well as the angle of the thrusting.

Q *Do you see the human need for sex as merely driven by biological impulses or are there other factors, such as a psychological need for intimacy, involved?*

A There are a few different things which you have mentioned that you are lumping into one question. Sex is considered, by some, as an expression of "life force energy". We are born as sexual beings, by the reality of our bodies, meaning we have innate sexual desires. Just because we have sexual desires does not mean that: 1) we know what to do with these sexual impulses (i.e. sexual behaviour for the large part is learned behaviour); 2) it is always acted upon; 3) it has to be with another human. There is also sex in the form of being by oneself, commonly known as masturbation, where there is intimacy with self. However, to answer your question more plainly, yes, sex is not just driven by biological impulses but also involves other factors such as how societal messages (including the media), cultural programming, and familial expectations play out on one's thinking (psychology) and consequently behaviour.

Q *Why do you think sexual imagery is so prevalent in the media and yet for sex treated as such a taboo subject in our society? What accounts for this contradiction?*

Ⓐ Advertisers are fighting to get the attention of their audiences. There is a widespread belief that "sex sells". Sexual imagery in the media is prevalent because it first captures attention and then uses sexual connotation or imagery to sell their products or services. However, as consumers continue to be exposed to such imagery, they might actually become desensitised or "numb" to it. These pervasive sexual images may subconsciously become their reality (i.e. it is normal or preferred to look or dress like models).

A very simple reason why the discussions about the prevalence of sexual imagery and sexuality are distinct is because the former is fuelled by advertisers, while the latter is an issue which has many "voices"—including governments, religious bodies, schools, parents etc.—all of whom have different (and often opposing) views about the extent of which sexuality should be discussed or addressed and how publicly. Even within the government, there are ministries with very different mandates. For instance, the Ministry of Education might be hard-pressed to introduce sexuality education programmes that would be accepted in all schools, including religious ones; the Ministry of Social and Family Development (MFS) might promote family values; and the Health Promotion Board might emphasize safer sex practices. It becomes an issue of who is more effective (or louder) with the limited budgets they have. Just because these "voices" are not heard does not mean they do not exist. As a percentage, the amount put into governmentally funded projects is probably a drop in the bucket compared to the billions spent on advertising with sexual imagery.

Q *What, in your opinion, is a healthy view and culture that a person should have towards sex?*

A In your question, I'm assuming, "sex" is just referring to the sexual act. It really should be "sexuality". Healthy sexuality involves the conscious expression of our sexual energy in ways that enhance our self-esteem, physical health and emotional relationship(s). It is mutually beneficial and harms no one. Healthy sexuality includes the ability to decide what being sexual means to us; to pursue the sexual lifestyle we choose to be engaged in; to be educated and to get information on our sexuality; to make decisions about our bodies (including about contraception and abortion). It includes being free of persecution, condemnation, discrimination or societal intervention in private sexual behaviour, and to receive non-judgemental sexual health care.

Kegels: Squeeze, Hold, Release

Your way to sexual health

Have you heard of pelvic floor exercises? You may have learned about them from your aerobics instructor. Or perhaps your urologist was the one who ordered you to squeeze your butt cheeks together? Maybe your gynae was the one who asked you to attempt to tighten your vagina, or was it your anus?

I have news for you: They're all the same thing. This exercise is more commonly known as the Kegel exercise.

Named after Dr Arnold Kegel, the Kegel exercise consists of contracting and relaxing the muscles that form part of the pelvic floor. The muscles actually being squeezed are known as the pubococcygeus muscles (or PC muscles for short) at the pelvic floor.

There are many benefits to doing Kegels. For men and women, it helps strengthens pelvic floor muscles weakened due to ageing, from being overweight, or for those who have a chronic cough, or a genetic predisposition to weak connective tissue.

Women who experience pelvic organ prolapse or urine leakage due to pregnancy and childbirth benefit from doing Kegels. Also women who have persistent problems reaching orgasm find Kegels sensitise their pelvic muscles. For men, Kegels aids in better ejaculatory control and can help treat prostate pain and swelling.

To locate your PC muscles, imagine how it feels when

you need to pee, but for whatever reason (say you are in a meeting), you are unable to immediately do so. Or try to stop the flow of urine while you are actually using the bathroom. That's right! Those are the muscles. After contracting those muscles, use your mind to relax them, you should feel your pelvic floor move back down to the starting position.

I can simplify the "How" into three keywords:

Frequency If you have never done any Kegels before, chances are your muscles are not well developed. Use a "squeeze, hold, release" pattern. Do so for a minimum of three sets (10 times per set) daily. If you are doing them correctly, you should feel some slight "burn" or tiredness around your outer thigh.

Duration Within days, you should be able to build up from duration of one second up to three seconds. If you can get to a count of 10, even 15, seconds, repeating the "squeeze, hold, and release"—that would be excellent!

Intensity As your muscles become stronger—and you become more experienced with the exercises—this movement will be more pronounced. This is when you have the ability to not only contract on the surface level, but squeeze even further. Much like how bodybuilders who lift weights push themselves just that bit more, you can also do that for your pelvic region!

Kegel exercises can be done anytime, anywhere. They are easy to do and require no special equipment. There is no reason not to do them, considering the benefits to bladder and bowel control and also sexual function! Give it a try!

The Full Body Workout in the Bedroom
Get fit while doing the deed!

Have you ever heard people saying that sex is a great workout? Did you know that just 30 minutes of intercourse can burn up to 200 calories? Instead of getting fit to have better sex, how about having sex to get fitter? Here are some simple sex positions that up the challenge in the bedroom:

Humpty rabbit

In this position, the woman squats above the man and uses her PC muscles (the same muscles you squeeze to stop yourself from peeing) to "catch" his member and clench him tight from within. She may support herself by putting her hands anywhere on his body for support, before guiding herself up and down. This variation of the woman-on-top position allows her to have better control of the depth and pace of the penetration. On his part, the man may lift his head and contract his stomach muscles—effectively giving his abdomen a hard workout. He can let his hands wonder and caress his partner's body.

Aroused dragon

If you like to have standing up sex, and yet are of different heights, the woman may be forced to go on tip-toe or on one leg. This is where her killer high heels come in. Besides showing off those sexy calves, she can do a little catwalk, swirl, and wink as she parts her legs for you. This promises an encore—where she will be performing cartwheels in your mind—long after the deed. Don't be afraid to get a short stool or side table to ease the technical difficulties of penetrating her while also supporting her lower body.

Entwined snakes

Lie on your back, turn to one side, and in a semi-twist, drape one leg over him. He also lies on his side facing her. Holding on to her thigh or bottom, he pulls her towards him. This allows your legs to be intertwined. This is a wonderful position for eye-gazing, which can stroke the flames of passion and increases the intimacy between the two of you.

Rocking horse

Sit facing each other with your legs entwined. From there, stretch out your arms and hold each other around the wrists or forearms. Take turns pulling each other so you are gently rocking back and forth like a rocking horse. Remember, practice makes perfect. As you learn to become more comfortable with this pose, your abs will invariably become more toned and you will be able to hold this pose for a prolonged length of time.

Soaring eagle

He is on top. She spreads her legs wide open, and then arches her back and lifts her hips up off the bed—all this from beneath him. This position not just exercises her bottom and thighs, but also helps her achieve clitoral stimulation! She may wish to reach out so as to hold onto him for additional support. Who says that a woman should lie back and think of England? She may be below, but she is not out of the action!

Laughing monkeys

In this position, the man is sitting up while the woman is sitting on him. She holds onto his neck—for dear life— with her hands, leans back, and raises her legs in the air in a straddle; while he manoeuvres her back and forth. More challenging than rocking horse, this will work the woman's arms, stomach and legs. The man will tone his arms while moving the woman's body, and will strengthen his legs from the support he is providing to his partner.

I hope these creative positions will inspire you to get moving in the bedroom—and, more importantly, enjoy yourselves while getting more fit physically.

***

Worrying about what you are doing "right" and approaching sex as only something you do for your partner, rather than doing and focusing on what feels pleasurable for you all interrupt the possibility of great sex.

Trickier positions are not necessarily better. You don't need to be upside down, hanging from a lamp or doing something crazy to have great sex. The emotional connection such as through gazing into each other's eyes can rock his world more than any sexual position could.

The best sex position is the one that makes the couple feel comfortable and works for them. Having said that, the most common and comfortable position couples use seems to be the missionary position (guy-on-top position).

1. **For a quickie**

    You have a few minutes and you want it hot, quick and sexy! Try Wall Standing Sex where both partners are standing doing penetration. The female uses a wall to support herself while being penetrated. Tip: Bend your knees to change the angle of penetration. The guy may wish to intense the depth of penetration by holding up his partner's leg or legs.

2. **To have a baby**

    It is a common myth that some sex positions are better than others if you're trying to get pregnant. The best sex position has to be the one that works best for you. My tip to have a baby is to have lots of sex, and enjoy the process, including the infinite sexual positions one can be in.

3. **For pleasure/fun**

    We probably all know the woman on top position. How about the reverse cowgirl sex position? This happens when the woman is facing away from her partner, who is lying down. Embrace your more assertive side and buy yourself a lasso or whip! The actual use of it on your partner is optional. Don't forget to make an appropriate noise that goes something along the lines of "Ye-ha!"

Q *My wife says I penetrate too deep. What can I do?*

A The woman-on-top position is the best position as it allows her to control the depth and pace of penetration. Missionary is next provided that you follow her verbal cues or non-verbal signals in penetrating slowly. Doggie position tends to be deepest. Spend more time on foreplay. Besides increasing lubrication, her vagina actually expands and lengthens when she is truly aroused, which will feel like there is more room inside.

Sex Toys

Gizmos and what not

A vibrator is usually turned on and positioned over the clitoris as part of the outer play before penetrative sex. Most vibrators come with different speeds and settings. You may experiment with varying amounts of pressure and motion until you reach climax. Consider using a little water-based lube to make it more pleasurable. A vibrator can actually be used on a man as well during intercourse. For a man, pressing the vibrator to the penis, especially the underside, can help stimulate it to erection. During intercourse, it is possible to slip a small vibrator like an egg in during just about any face-to-face position, for instance between her outer labia and over the clitoris.

For starters, you can use a vibrating ring which looks like a hair band except it has an external battery with an on-off switch. Have the man stretch the vibrating ring over his penis and rest it at the base of his erect or non erect penis, and watch the penis come to life as you turn the ring on. Ride him as you usually do and the added stimulation may well help you get a stronger orgasm. If he isn't comfortable with a vibration ring at the base of his penis, you can always use the vibrating ring for outer play such as on your clitoris or around your vulva. The best thing about vibrating rings is that you can buy them readily at Watsons or Guardian outlets without needing to step into a sex shop.

If you are open to go to a sex shop, ask the shop assistant what they would recommend a lady as a first sex toy.

- Do you want it for external stimulation or internal?
- Does the look matter? Or the colour?
- How about the intensity?
- Or the types of vibrations you can get out of it?
- Would it be more value for money for you if it was waterproof?

Have a think before you go in. I usually recommend ladies getting their first sex toy to get something small, discreet and pretty, such as a "bullet" which looks basically like a small egg attached to a wire which leads to a controller. Once you have a positive experience with your first sex toy, you can always go back to the shop and ask for other recommendations. Lastly, go to a friendly, sex-positive and non-pushy sex shop such as U4Ria in Singapore. I have recommended all my clients to them because of the above-mentioned reasons and many reported having had positive experiences, including the extremely shy ladies.

Technology-related

Q *Regarding your view of technological implements such as sex toys in its use to facilitate sexual experiences. Do you think that engaging in "sex" with certain sex toys such as blow-up dolls is a healthy practice?*

A What is healthy? Who decides? When does what is "healthy" become "unhealthy"? For example, when does one know one has eaten too much of a particular indulgence, say, chocolate? What can we say about a society that condones over-eating, but acts all phobic when it comes to pleasure of a different kind? Could it be that the negative publicity about sex is a result of ignorance and lack of any real understanding of sexuality at large? How does the use of "certain" sex toys hurt anybody? And why is what is a personal choice any of anybody's business? To answer your question simply, certainly, the incorporation of sex toys into one's sexual life can only enhance the experience, and is, thence, healthy and positive.

Q *Does it diminish the human-to-human nature of sexual experiences?*

A First of all, sex toys are not always used in isolation, but are also incorporated during partnered sex.

Just as with anything, it is about being aware of the sensations within your own body. Do not persist on using your sex toys if your body is sore, hurting or just "had enough" for the day. Our body is capable of learning and re-learning different ways to have pleasure.

Q *How has the rise of the Internet and mass media changed people's perceptions or sex and sexual behaviour?*

A The increased use of the Internet has allowed surfers to easily seek sexual information, knowledge, education as well as gratification online.

Q *Do you feel that such advances dehumanise sex?*

A What is sex? What is dehumanising? Who decides? We are not in kindergarten anymore, where decisions are made for us by adults around us. Being an adult means being able to decide for ourselves how we like to express our sexuality and to be free to pursue our sexual desires—including the use of sexual aids and with the help of technology.

Q *For example, technology facilitating sexual experiences in a virtually simulated environment?*

A We already live in what can be described as a virtually simulated environment. There is the television, iPhone, iPad, Internet, online sex chat forums, webcam sex, sexting, etc.

Q *My girlfriend wants me to use a vibrator on her. Does it mean I'm inadequate?*

A Many people believe that "real sex" has to be somehow without any outside influence (no lubricant, no sex toys, etc.). Using vibrators is a completely healthy and pleasurable way to explore your sexuality. Common reasons people play with vibrators include curiosity, self-discovery, to spice up a long-term relationship, for fun, to experience orgasm for the first time, or for extra stimulation that you can't add on your own. Expand your mind and shift your beliefs. A vibrator will never replace the emotion and intimacy possible with another person.

Think of the vibrator as your representative, ally or extra pair of hands and enjoy!

Q *I have a healthy sex life with my husband. Why do I still need sex toys? How can it improve my situation?*

A It is no secret that a few novelty items can spice up any sexual relationship—making a good one, better! Sex toys are no longer as taboo a subject as they once were. There are shops that carry anything from sexy lingerie to sex toys which can be ordered by online.

Vibrators can enhance your pleasure during self or partner play, to arouse you as a warm-up to your usual intimacies, to help you achieve orgasm or have multiple orgasms, and even to provide a great back massage. With a vibrator, you can be pleasured for as long as you wish and best of all, you are in the driver's seat.

Many women experience stronger, more intense orgasms with a vibrator's consistent stimulation. Regular orgasms have been proven to boost your immune system and keep your pelvic floor muscles strong and toned. So vibrators can help you have better health!

Sexting as a form of foreplay

- Your teasing can help build up the suspense and lead to hot wild in-person sex.
- Your imagination is free to go wild. Half the fun is imagining the face of your partner upon reading your naughty thoughts. Lighten up! Sex is supposed to be fun!

- If you are still in the flirting stage, it can help you to ease your way to the next step.
- Removes some of the embarrassment you might feel otherwise face-to-face. It keeps you on your toes, thinking of new things to say and new ways to respond.

Dos and don'ts of sexting?
Do

- Delete your conversation when you're done playing. Never use your work phone.
- Ask or test the waters before you are sure he or she is into it.
- Take it slowly. Pace yourself and follow your partner's lead. You'll know what feels right and what doesn't.
- Choose someone you trust. Need I say more?
- Use some humour and inside jokes.
- Send an appropriate smiley face from time to time to let your partner know all is well!

Don't

- Send your sex message to the wrong person!
- Sext someone you've just met. Sexting cannot be used as a way to pick up a partner. Texting is fine. Sexting is not.
- Engage in textual intercourse with multiple partners at the same time.
- Forget to clean your room before trying to be sexy on

camera. It can defeat the whole point of what you are
trying to achieve.

• Sexting is really just another way to communicate.
It's a fun, easy way to express yourself and to test the
boundaries of how or what you should talk to your
partner about.

Q *How can women or men protect themselves from getting into
trouble over sexting i.e. having their photos splashed online?*

A The only foolproof way to protect yourself is this: don't
do it. It may seem like a good idea at the time, but once a
photo is out there, you can't get it back. It's better to tell
your partner to use his or imagination.

Don't include your face in the photos. There is no
guarantee it will not appear in cyberspace. A scorned lover
can go to extreme means to make your life miserable.
Promises can be broken. You always have a choice to
not engage in sexting at all. It may be better to tell your
partner to use his or imagination. The other way is to
engage in sexting within self imposed limits—for instance
not including sexually suggestive photographs.

Fantasy
When it is in the head

Fantasising is normal

Your mind is your most powerful sex organ, and your skin is your largest one! The brain programmes our sexual functionality, our reproductive behaviour, and sets the boundaries of our sex drive. Hence, it has the potential to be our most powerful tool for accessing better, mind-blowing (literally!) sex. This applies for both men and women.

Fantasising can stay in your head

We can use our minds to fantasise about anything—even the impossible or seemingly unattainable. Fantasies are healthy and normal as long as you can separate them from reality and accept (and sometimes appreciate) that you may not be able to fulfil them. What goes on in your mind stays in your mind. For many, fantasies should remain the way they are—fantasies—as reality creates potential for let-down. You should not feel you need to share your fantasies with your partner especially if he or she is not going to be receptive or open to this and will be hurt.

Fantasizing is okay

In fact, I would say don't be afraid to "get yourself ready" for sex through fantasy. Desire might not always occur spontaneously, especially if you are tired or stressed. Give yourself permission to use your sexual imagination.

Sharing your fantasies

We want to feel that our desires are normal and acceptable. Because you love your spouse, his or her opinion of your sexual desires and fantasies play a bigger role than you might realise. While you should not let her make you feel uncomfortable, remember that you should not make a loved one feel odd or uncomfortable by insisting on imposing either. Sharing your fantasies may well bring both of you closer—or alienate your partner depending on *how* you approach the subject— openly, honestly, jokingly, warmly, with clear differentiation between fantasy and reality, and no pressure on him or her to accept your fantasy.

Fantasising is not about forcing your partner to do anything

In any kind of partnered sex, this is all about finding the middle ground with what works and feels good for both of you. As such, sex is not just about doing what your partner wants and giving it to the other person. It is also about what you want and what makes you feel good.

If you persist on pushing your boundaries and being disrespectful of your partner's desires, this will not work out well. It is important to recognise that we have multiple roles in our lives—parent, child, mother, wife or career person. Sharing fantasies can also be fun, liberating and very intimate, and only possible because of existing trust, openness and a willingness to be vulnerable.

***

Women are just as capable as men of using porn sex to perk up their sex lives. A fantasy which she might like to re-enact is how she is so desirable to her partner that he cannot stop himself from ravishing her and "using" her for sex.

These are some gross generalisations but off the top of my head, they would include:

For men: threesome; anal sex on the woman; cumming in her mouth, chest, and the like.

For women: romanticised sex e.g. candles, music, silk bedsheets, roses and the like; being raped.

Q *From a woman: what happens if you fantasise about lots of things to do in bed—but in reality, you're shy. You worry he'll think the idea is silly e.g. role play. How can you be more adventurous, and minimise the risk of rejection?*

A To lose your inhibitions during sex, one idea is to ask your lover if you can use a blindfold. Since your partner cannot see you, it will help you feel much less inhibited and more confident, which allows you to engage in sexual activities you wouldn't otherwise. For instance, you could try a genital massage, new sexual position or sex toy. Just use plenty of lube for a smoother and sexier experience.

A blindfold heightens sensation, increases psychological vulnerability, but also adds an element of surprise.

- Create your blindfold from scarves, ties or handkerchiefs you can get hold of.

- Spice things up by feeding your lover delectable items.
- Combine some light bondage by tying your beau's wrists to some part of your headboard or tie them together over his head or behind his back.

Erotica

When reading is foreplay

In an age where porn is so easily accessible on the Internet and on our smartphones, what do you think is the appeal of reading erotic books or steamy book passages?

These are the possible benefits of erotica:

1. The steamy sex scenes in erotic literature can be very much more interesting because you are the one making up your own visuals!
2. Erotica can help fuel your imagination, not to mention creativity in the bedroom.
3. Reading them to each other can aid sexual arousal.
4. Not only could new interests be discovered when doing such reading, erotica can act as a stimulus for more open communication about sex—and what might work for each other.
5. Men are more inclined to feel entitled to masturbate, but women often do not. Erotica can help women who have inhibitions to fan their desire first before proceeding further, whether in solo sex or with a partner.
6. And then there is the possibility of role playing in one's body or enacting a scene with a partner.

Most women find the images in porn videos disgusting and that porn is overtly focused on the end result of orgasm/ejaculation. Is there an argument that erotic fiction is more "female-friendly" or appeals more to female sensibilities?

1. **Shift in perspective.** Erotica helps women park their roles of mother, wife, employer or employee on the back burner and connect with their sexual, juicy, adventurous selves. Reading a satisfying love scene stirs a woman's emotions, which are directly linked to her libido. Bibliotherapy helps women to tune in, turn on… and experience a more intimate and satisfying sexual relationship with their partner and themselves!

2. **Naughtiness in the head.** Women often would never do what they actually fantasise about. Reading about outrageous sexual behaviour they can imagine about is a terrific way to stir up all sorts of newfound naughtiness in the bedroom. In creating or expanding into a zone of permission, fun and lightness, women can learn to share and experience sensuality and pleasure on a deeper, more primal level.

3. **I never thought of that!** Erotic authors know how the female primal brain works and what turns them on. Their stories will give delicious new ideas women want to try at home—things they would never have in a million years thought of themselves!

4. **More fun, more open** *Psychology Today* states that women who read romance novels make love with their

partners 74% more often than women who don't. And according to *The Journal of Sex Research,* when women fantasize frequently (as they do when they read erotic novels), they have sex more often, have more fun in bed, and engage in a wider variety of erotic activities.

5. **A happy break.** Erotica bring women into a world of happy endings and steamy adventures when they need respite from all the doom and gloom of their daily newspapers and other stuff that will only leave them feeling slightly depressed and perpetually exhausted? So what if one escapes from life occasionally? The benefits are real and valuable, and the emotional gratification received will spill into their own relationship.

Porn
Larger-than-life sex

Both men and women can get turned on by things they can see. Considering that their arousal is usually linked to images, most men would have masturbated to pictures of female bodies from their teens.

Many men use porn for quick masturbation—and this can happen even if they are in a sexually satisfying relationship. When men masturbate, they tend to be very task-orientated in getting the orgasmic release and "relief" so that they can relax or sleep better. To many men, porn is compartmentalised into being an "extra" in their lives, or even a tool or aid for sexual arousal and eventual orgasm. In general, men do not view porn or solo sex as a sign of infidelity.

It is thus not surprising that porn images and portrayals become embedded as part of their thought patterns, fantasies, dreams and even subconscious mind. Therefore many people, at some point in their lives with the right partner, would like to portray porn sex. That, by itself, is not harmful.

Word about porn: There is absolutely nothing "unhealthy" or abnormal with watching porn in and of itself. As long as they are legal adult movies, and where everyone involved including those who are watching are consenting, there is nothing inherently bad in pornography; that would be akin to saying sex is bad. Keep in mind that *not* everybody who watch porn do so in unhealthy ways, watch too much of it or become obsessive about it.

Do you think porn is unhealthy and damaging to a couple's sex life?

No. As with anything, it depends how you approach it. I do not see porn sex by itself as harmful if it's between two mutually consenting adults who are able to recognise porn sex as one of the options in their sexual toolkit repertoire and occasionally engage in such activity. The harm can happen when either partner is distressed about the style of lovemaking or is getting frustrated or bored with being objectified. This is when an honest dialogue should take place.

The reality is that porn is having a profound impact on our culture. Rather than argue about the harmful effects of porn, it might be far more worthwhile discussing its specific effects on your relationship (and there are many), then recognise ways to navigate those better.

On performance anxiety

Most porn sex can actually lead to men having a degree of performance anxiety since not all men have huge penises, are capable of having sex for a long time or climax again and again. They might compare themselves against porn actors, feel inadequate and become perpetually unsatisfied with their own bodies and sexual performance.

The other way of looking at porn sex is at how the male actor is always the star as well as initiator and aggressor. Men can identify with or model the porn actors by tapping into their inner performer or "star". To do so would require emotionally distancing himself from the act and spectatoring

to some degree ('How am I doing?" vs. "How does she feel?").
This fixation with performance could also "short-circuit" his
actually being present in the experience and enjoying the
sexual experience. Hence a man who "performs" better in bed
may not necessarily be a good lover in terms of meeting his
partner's emotional, sexual and intimacy needs.

Why or why not?

Not all porn are made the same. If you approach porn with
the right attitude: that it is essentially entertainment and
therefore may not depict reality, and are using it for whatever
value it brings i.e. as a visual stimuli,

Q *Can watching porn together really spice things up?*

A Her negative attitude of porn comes from how most flicks
portray women only as sex subjects for the gratification
of their partner. Porn also goes against her belief that sex
should only be between two people in love. Reassure her
of your love, and that watching porn together is just for
sexual inspiration. An easier transition is if you start with
amateur porn or porn made by women for women online.

Q *What is porn addiction, clinically speaking?*

A Porn consumption is not necessarily or inescapably wrong
so long as it's legal adult movies, and where everyone who
is watching is consenting. Porn can become a problem
when you can't get off without it. You want to watch for
if it is interfering with your sexual expectations, distorting

your conception of real women and real bodies, causing issues in your relationship, or making you not feel good but you use it anyways. If you are concerned about being reliant on porn, then you may wish to work with a trained sexologist or sex therapist to discuss your concerns.

Porn Sex

Q *How common is it for men to be inspired by porn flicks in the bedroom?*

A In December 2009, a Canadian study sought to compare the views of 20-something men who watch porn with those who didn't. They ran into a problem: they couldn't find a *single* man who hadn't seen porn. Closer to home, according to The Porn Report, up to one third of Australian adults consume some kind of pornography ever year, and for over 99% of them it's just a small part of their lives. Hence it is not surprising that some of the most common sexual fantasies and inspiration to lovemaking that men have are derived from porn.

Q *What exactly is "porn sex"? What sorts of things does it mean he will be doing? Will he try to be more adventurous in bed?*

A Porn sex happens when men or women begin re-enacting what happens in porn in the bedroom, sometimes subconsciously or unintentionally. This could be from repeating what porn stars say "Take it baby", objectifying a woman or being objectified as a woman where all sex ends with the male orgasm, to wanting the "money shot" where sex ends in the face of the woman.

It is just that the ubiquity of porn has blurred the line between screen and life, acting and reality, performance sex and lovemaking. Porn has "distorted" the ideas men think of what sex is and the ways young males think about sex. This doesn't mean that role-playing or imaging yourself to be a porn star cannot be fun or arousing if taken in the right spirit.

Q *Would he expect his women to act in a certain way in the bedroom?*

A He might assume it is acceptable to ejaculate on his partner's face or breasts. This sort of material is common in porn, leading many men to think this is routine behaviour in the bedroom. In fact, I have heard of ignorant couples who do not realise that that is not how you get pregnant.

Q *What advice would you give to women who are bored of the "porn sex" and want to change it up?*

A The first step would be to discuss openly with her partner her boredom with porn sex, and to include specific suggestions for change. This might include agreeing on what type of porn and how much porn can be viewed. Alternative forms of media are porn by women for women or sex education videos that can often be arousing as well as informative.

If she wishes to stay away from any kind of sexually explicit media, she could enrol her partner and herself into the various sexual enhancement or enrichment classes to expand their sexual skills and knowledge. She could also consider engaging the services of a clinical sexologist to learn practical yet meaningful ways to "shake" up her sex life or exercises that can build intimacy in relationships.

People often find it difficult to communicate about anything related to sex, but it is necessary to recognise that communication is key in any relationship. If you avoid discussing issues until it becomes a problem, talking may no longer be effective.

Mindful Sex

Have you ever felt glad, relieved even, to get away from someone because the person would not stop talking, and worse yet, about themselves?

Have you wished the person sitting behind you on the bus or standing behind you on the train would stop talking into their phone or to the person next to them at the top of their voice?

Then there is the gym. Have you ever wondered just why personal trainers need to be yelling when their client is just next to them, at the expense of everybody else there?

When I go the gym, there is loud techno-thumping music blasting from the speakers overhead. It is so loud that in order to override it, I would have to turn my preferred music on my headset to its full volume. On the rare occasions when I am the first at the gym, I ask them to kindly turn the music down, only to have it back up during my next visit.

Silence is how we hear ourselves think. It is how we can listen to that still, small voice, also known as our inner voice, speak to us. Silence is how we catch our breath, process our thoughts, decipher our wishes and make decisions. Sometimes, I hear of people who are afraid of silence, afraid of being by themselves, afraid of facing the truth.

Apparently it is so difficult to find silence that it is now a commodity. According to the New York Post in 2010, you can experience a weeklong silent retreat at Shreyas Spa in Bangalore, India for US$3,000. A bargain compared to the US$21,000 that the Canadian Health Ministry shelled out for 15 bureaucrats to spend two days and one night in the countryside not speaking to one another.

Living in a highly urbanised and densely populated place is no joke. There is no respite, no escape, and no room to breathe other than into the armpit of your fellow commuter.

Find pockets of time, go within and be silent. In recent weeks, I have learned that there are other ways to meditate besides sitting cross-legged and being still.

For instance, there is:

- Laughing meditation. Visit my MeetUp group
  www.meetup.com/singaporelaughteryoga/
- Movement meditation. Check out Oneness Flow
  www.onenessflow.com
- Writing meditation. Do morning pages and weekly
  reflections with the book, *The Artist's Way at Work*.

You may question just how laughing, moving or writing can be meditative. If you do it for the sake of doing it, then it is just activity or busyness. If, however, you engage in an activity and are completely absorbed by it, could care less what others think and are truly enthralled with the here and now, that is meditation. That is when your problems disappear. For that brief moment, the world fades away, and you exist. Be silent and know it is ok to be still.

Seeking Mind-blowing Sex

It goes without saying that what is mind-blowing sex to me may not be such for you. Also, what works sexually for me might not work for others. So, how can one actually define what is "the best" sex or "great" sex? Apparently, some brave scientists have attempted to answer this age-old question.

In 2010, Peggy Kleinplatz at the University of Ottawa and A. Dana Ménard of Carleton University found six major themes of what makes for "great sex" or optimal sexuality. These may be the building blocks toward the farther reaches of human erotic potential and consist of: being present, authenticity, intense emotional connection, sexual and erotic intimacy, communication, and transcendence.

Ponder upon them so that you might be closer to your goal on your path to nirvana.

Being present

The most predominant and fully articulated characteristic of great sex was of being "fully present" and "totally absorbed in the moment." One is definitely not thinking of work, checking off the To-do list for the day or worrying about the kids. You are just enjoying each moment for what it is, including all the sensations running through your body.

Authenticity

This refers to the ability of being themselves, feeling free to be themselves with their partners, and being relentlessly honest with themselves. The very act of being honest and open to one's own desires is freeing and energising, as well as powerful. When one is open and increasing in self-knowledge, the opportunities for self-growth also increase. Participants could not have said it better in sharing: "Sexual encounters provide a unique and treasured opportunity for growth, for welcoming of unknowns, with the partner acting as a catalyst to affect self discovery."

Intense emotional connection

Whether in long-term or other relationships, all great sex involved a powerful sense of intimate engagement. All participants stated that intense emotional contact for the duration of the encounter was an integral aspect of great sex. The degree of connection, energy, "alignment" or "conductivity" between the persons all determined how great the sex could be. This includes having trust, cherishing one another, sharing, accepting, validating, and feeling "as much desired as desiring".

Sexual and erotic intimacy

This relates to the importance of a deep sense of caring for one another, regardless of the duration of the relationship. Intimacy was seen as making an exponential difference. Sexual intimacy was predicated on an emotional bond, and was seen as instrumental in sexual bonding.

Communication

For most participants, great sex required excellent communication, and was seen as crucial to the success of a sexual encounter. They spoke in terms of the abilities to listen, respond, being able to give and to receive feedback, to be non-judgemental, to organise information and having the ability to give positive regard, thereby, "making people inspired to give back more". There was also the ability to read the partner's response via one's own body, specifically via touch.

Transcendence

Great sex appears to involve a combination of heightened altered mental, emotional, physical, relational and spiritual states in unison. This meant being awash in "awe", "ecstasy", "bliss", "peace", and "the sublime". Sexual intercourse was regarded as a metaphor for the "ultimate form of merging".

Home assignment

- Share this chapter with your partner and discuss which of the above areas are working for you and which ones could be improved.
- Brainstorm about what could make your sex life sizzle more.
- Decide on one option and agree on a date and time to carry out your idea.
- Carry out, evaluate and re-strategise. Have fun!

Older, Wiser and Still Sexual

Have you ever heard of the expressions "dirty old man" or "little old lady"? These negative stereotypes are reinforced by sexuality among older people being seldom portrayed or discussed. As age catches up, you find yourself having a few wrinkles, getting grey and gaining weight. However, the desire for sexual contact can remain high and even unchanged. The first step in continuing to be sexual is to understand the kinds of physical changes and psychological effects of ageing and what you can do about them.

Physical changes

The most common cause for changes in the level of sexual desire for both men and women is attributed to testosterone or oestrogen hormonal imbalance. A health check is in order. In addition, there are health conditions that can decrease sexual interest and behaviours such as: high blood pressure, arthritis, menopause, depression, pulmonary diseases, diabetes, incontinence, and coronary artery disease. A common side effect of many medications for these conditions is the inhibition of sexual desire. It is important to have an honest discussion with your doctor about any negative side effect arising from your medications.

Psychological effects

Partners may become physically and personally less attractive to each other for all sorts of reasons, not just due to ageing. Negative thoughts, feelings or emotions reduce the interest in sex. Traumatic or sad experiences that have not been dealt with, like the loss of a partner, can influence sexual desire negatively. Stress, irrational thoughts, relational problems are some other causes. Differences in sexual needs and the refusal of partners to respond to advances can lead to doubts about self-image.

Suggestions:

1. Endeavour to take better care of yourself. A self-care programme includes good nutrition combined with effective and regular exercise. Hormone replacement therapy for hormonal imbalance is an option.

2. For women, when pelvic floor muscle strength starts to slip (which is accelerated by loss of oestrogen), you may begin to feel as though "nothing happens down there anymore". Exercise your pelvic floor to maintain your connection with the experience of sexual arousal. Tension of the pelvic floor is critical to most people's experience of "feeling turned on".

3. In the rush of everyday life, sex very often doesn't include time for a warm-up. Accept that you may need more time for arousal. Snuggles, gentle caresses and physical intimacy are important to a woman. By losing some of the focus on the orgasm, older men can achieve

a great deal of pleasure from sexual intimacy. Then there is expanding your sexual repertoire, such as oral sex, manual sex, mutual masturbation, sex toys, etc. These can aid in attaining stronger erections and orgasms.

4. Use it or lose it. When you have an orgasm, the contractions bring blood flow to your pelvis, helps keep your tissues strong and thick, and your pelvic muscles strong and flexible. It also utilises your circulatory system and your nervous system, and helps keep everything running smoothly. Having regular orgasms (at least one per week) helps keep these muscles in shape, and reminds your body how to "do" sexual arousal. A vibrator can speed up the process if you wish.

5. You deserve the best quality of care. So take ownership of your sexuality by developing awareness of body changes, asking your doctor questions and getting accurate information. A sexologist can help address your sexual concerns, including how to modify your sexual techniques so as to continue having pleasure from sex. Sex plays an important role in your sense of well-being. The sexual experience enhances emotional attachment and facilitates intimacy in our relationships. You may be older and wiser, but you are also definitely capable of remaining sexual. There is no age limit on sex.

APPENDIX
36 Things I Wish I Learned in Sex Ed

Growing up in a relatively typical Chinese family in Singapore, I received very little sexuality education. Let me give you the context: I did not know that what I had "down there" was called the vulva even though I had the "bits". I did not attempt to pronounce the word "penis" until I was 26, and as if that by itself was not awkward enough, I was then told that I said it wrong!

Here are nine things that I wish I had learned in sex-ed as a teenager:

1. The correct anatomical names for the genitals. Without knowing what is "down there" and resorting to using pet names or blushing every time we refer to our private parts, just how comfortable can one be with one's sexuality, much less sexual expression? Being able to give the correct anatomical names to your genitals is part of healthy sexuality.

2. Adults do not talk to you about sex because they are afraid of being responsible for telling you the wrong things about sex, but mostly it is because they are uncomfortable talking about sex themselves. Forgive them for never being able to give you a straight answer or dismissing you because they still see you as a child. Let that go.

3. Do not believe everything you hear from your friends,
    family or anybody else for that matter about sex. Most
    of the time, they are just passing on what they heard
    from somebody, who heard it from somebody else.

4. It is okay to seek out information about sex and
    sexuality. It does not make you any less of a person,
    but instead better prepared to make the right sexual
    decisions for YOU. The more you actually do know
    about sex and sexuality, the more comfortable you will
    be in owning and expressing your sexuality. Sex is not
    dirty, but rather completely natural and normal.

5. Sexuality education does not encourage the early start of
    sexual intercourse, the frequency of intercourse, or even
    an increase in the number of sexual partners among the
    young. Instead, understanding sexuality can actually
    delay the onset of intercourse, reduce the frequency of
    intercourse, reduce the number of sexual partners, and
    increase condom or contraceptive use.

6. Sexuality education has very little to do with the
    sexual act, but is actually a lifelong process of
    acquiring information and forming the attitudes,
    beliefs and values of one's sexuality. It encompasses
    sexual development, sexual and reproductive health,
    interpersonal relationships, affection, intimacy, body
    image and gender roles.

7. Our desire for sex is natural, but the act of sex itself is learned. Like much of everything we know, we acquire the knowledge, practise it through trial and error, and perfect it so that it becomes a skill which we "own". Hence, the phrase: "sexual skill". Sex is a skill. You may still benefit from attending sexual workshops when you grow up.

8. Though it can be for some people, sex is not just a physical act. Sex is usually a physical, emotional, mental and even spiritual act. Your intention has everything to do with what sex is like for you.

9. Your skin is your biggest sex organ, and your brain is your most powerful sex organ. Use both, and let go of any guilt! Enjoy your body, enjoy being alive, and breathe! Give yourself permission to use your sexual imagination. Your sexual fantasies, desires and dreams are valuable and integral parts of your sexuality.

The only sexuality education I received in secondary school (or high school in the US) was in the form of annual school talks presented by pharmaceutical companies promoting sanitary pads or tampons (depending where they were from). The boys got to first jeer at us, as they went out to play in the sun. We, the young ladies, had the burden of listening to instruction on menstruation and the need to clean up after ourselves.

10. There needs to always be authentic consent for sex to happen. Silence is not consent. Drunken sex is not consent. Consent can be withdrawn at any time. It is okay to stop a sexual session or leave if you do not feel it is right or good for you.

11. There is a difference between being coerced to doing something and being curious and open-minded for your own sake. Heard of the saying, "Fake it till you make it?" Sometimes all it takes to get used to something new is doing more of it so that you get used to it. For instance, it may include getting used to the look, smell and taste of his penis and even semen.

12. Rather than let sex happen to you, begin thinking about what you need for sex to happen. What would make sex good for you? What would make it better? The first thing is to know what it is you want.

13. You have the right to ask about the sexual history of your partner; whether what they tell you is true or not is another matter. Always choose safer sex practices. Take charge; purchase and carry protection with you.

14. Worry less about pleasing your partner and more about doing the right thing by you—things that after doing you can live to face yourself in the mirror the next day.

Remember, it is your body, your life and your future that is on the line. Before you can have any kind of meaningful relationship, first recognise the magnificence within you and love yourself.

15. Sexual communication is communication. You probably already have the skills it takes to ask for what you need and want sexually. Because your desires and preferences may change over time, sexual communication must be an ever-evolving process. You deserve the best sex possible so communicate.

16. Sex involves the expression of physical love. It is about the joy of life as well as the intimacy of connectedness. The intimacy that these couples must have has to do with the ability to share one's fears, dreams and pains. Without honesty, patience and the ability to be vulnerable, it is not possible to let your partner know who you really are and what you really want.

17. Masturbation is sex. Foreplay is sex. Oral sex is sex. Anal sex is sex. Penis in the vagina is sex. The lack of the male or female orgasm is still sex. To a sexologist, there are different forms of sexual expressions and once one enters the sexual response cycle, it counts as sex! And there is nothing wrong with the word sex either!

18. There is a difference between fantasy and reality. In our fantasies, there are no repercussions, no harm, or pain physically felt or experienced. Fantasies are stimulating because they would probably not happen in real life. This does not mean fantasies cannot become reality, nor does it mean that all fantasies should be played out in life. What is more important is that you can separate between fantasy and reality, and are able to decide what you wish to retain as a fantasy, and what you would like to have happen down the road and under what circumstances.

I was probably 11 or 12 when I watched a video called "The Silent Scream" in primary school (or grade school in the US). It is a documentary that depicts the abortion process via ultrasound and shows an abortion taking place in the uterus. During the abortion process, the presenter dramatically paused the video as the 11-week fetus opens its mouth in the uterus—in what appeared to be an outcry of pain and discomfort—and went, "There, there, there is the silent scream!"

Satisfied that we are considerably traumatised, we were each left with a silver collar pin moulded after the feet of an 11-week foetus to remind us of the consequences if we were to have sex. From what I hear, generations of students have watched this video in Singapore. This singular video was the only form of sex ed I can remember in primary school.

19. All these things your doctor or parents told you is all is true: watch your diet, exercise regularly, drink less, stop smoking, and take time to pamper yourself. Your ability to enjoy your sexuality is in direct correlation with your general health.

20. You do not end up with a shorter life, go blind, or develop hairy palms from performing masturbation. There are lots of nice alternative names for masturbation such as self-love, self-pleasuring or even solo-sex which you can choose to use.

21. If you are unable to achieve an orgasm by yourself, you are less likely to be able to have an orgasm with a partner. Understanding your own body through masturbation is a great way to express your sexuality, to relieve stress and to sleep better.

22. Most women (70–80%) can only attain an orgasm through clitoral stimulation. Only about 10–20% of women can reach an orgasm through vaginal penetration. An orgasm is an orgasm is an orgasm. There is no good or bad way to receive an orgasm, so just enjoy!

23. Because men experience the start of their orgasm and ejaculation contractions within a fraction of a second, it is often misunderstood (even by the media) as one

and the same thing. In reality, men can orgasm without ejaculating, and men can also ejaculate without an orgasm.

24. Yes, there is such a thing called the female G-spot. There is also the male G-spot, and E-spot (where arousal happens as the ear is being cleaned). It is also true that some women can ejaculate and it is not pee though it may contain traces of urine. Instead of being stuck on locating "spots", what is most important is that you are experiencing pleasure and enjoying yourself during sex.

25. While the mass media uses sexualised images of men and women to sell their products and services, the people depicted do not represent how the rest of the population actually looks. Rather than be fixated with weight, focus on health. Instead of getting caught up with looking like a model, concern yourself with the beauty you hold within and let it shine through. It will serve you well.

26. While porn always ends with the male orgasm, sex in real life does not need to end that way. The goal of sex should not be the orgasm. Either or both or neither one of you might "cum" in any given sexual encounter and that is alright!

27. While watching porn, it is important to remember that they are actors portraying what most people fantasise about, not what actually happens in most people's sex lives. That aside, we can be sexually stimulated by a wide variety of music, art, pictures, movies, stories, etc. and it is not at all weird if you do too.

One does not set out to be a sexuality educator, not one coming from a typical Chinese family anyway. I became one to help people because I was tired of sex always being talked about in negative ways.

28. Alcohol may relax you. Alcohol may make you perform better sexually. But alcohol also numbs sensation and pleasure and inhibits judgement.

29. If you experience pain when engaging in self pleasuring, when performing oral sex on somebody, or when giving or receiving penetrative sex (vaginal or anally), slow down or stop! Always listen to your body!

30. If we listen to the signals our body sends us, why do we not listen to what our heart tells us? When we become better at identifying and expressing our emotional feelings, we become more socially adept at establishing and building relationships. The more socially adept we become, the better we feel and the better our relationships will be.

31. We get caught up with what is "normal", "correct", and "acceptable." It dominates our thinking on everything from length and size of anatomical parts, to sexual frequency, duration and positioning. Especially in sex, there is actually no such thing called "normal".

32. Always regard negative statistics and studies relating to sex and sexuality with a pinch of salt. Such reports are only as accurate as the quality of their sample and manner in which the study was conducted, and sometimes by whom it was funded. They do not necessarily represent the rest of the world and, most likely, they do not represent you.

33. Modern science tells us that homosexuality is a human variation, not a mental illness and, therefore, has no need for a cure. One's sexual orientation has no bearing on their value system or the quality of their character. Homosexuals are perfectly capable of being faithful and forming happy and long lasting relationships.

34. Discount negative media portrayals of queer people. These stereotypical images are used to help move the plot along quickly. Instead view ALL humans as unique individuals with varied sexual desires, needs and wants, who may choose to express their sexuality in ways that society may not consider "normal". (But remember, there is no such thing as "normal".)

35. Your relationship with sex and your sexuality will change, and sometimes that change is on a daily basis. For instance, for post-pregnancy women, some parts will change. Beyond accepting and understanding the changes of your body is to work with what you have.

36. It is common to experience some form of sexual anxiety in your life. Should you be distressed and your condition has not changed in six months, you may wish to seek professional support.

Resources for people interested in sex and sexuality in Singapore

- **Action for AIDS** (AfA)
  http://www.afa.org.sg
- **DSC Clinic**
  The DSC (Department of Sexually Transmitted Infections Control) Clinic is a specialist outpatient clinic for the diagnosis, treatment and control of STIs in Singapore. http://www.dsc-sexualhealth.com.sg/
- **AWARE Singapore**
  Focuses on women's rights
  http://www.aware.org.sg
- **Health Xchange**
  Singapore's Trusted Health & Lifestyle Portal.
  http://www.healthxchange.com.sg

GLBT

- **Sayoni** is a community of queer women who organise and advocate for equality regardless of sexual orientation and gender identity.
  http://www.sayoni.com/
- **People Like Us 3 (PLU3)**
  http:// www.plu.sg/society
- **Adventurers Like Us (ADLUS)**
  http://sgwiki.com/wiki/Singapore_LGBT_organisations

Sexual health stes

- **The New School of Erotic Touch**

  The largest and most beautiful collection of explicit erotic massage educational video found anywhere on the web.
  http://tinyurl.com/nf4qkqe

- **Scarleteen**

  Real, up-to-date explicit information about sex and sexuality written clearly for teens.
  http://www.scarleteen.com/

- **Sexetc.org**

  Sponsored by the Network for Family Life Education, Rutgers University.
  http://sexetc.org/

- **Sexuality Information and Education Council of the United States (SIECUS)**

  http://www.siecus.org/

- **Society for Human Sexuality**

  This is a list of resources and some great articles.
  http://www.sexuality.org/

- **San Francisco Sex Information (SFSI)**

  http://sfsi.org/

- **NetDoctor**

  UK's leading independent health website.
  http://www.netdoctor.co.uk/

Acknowledgements

My gratitude…

- To Melvin Neo, managing editor at Marshall Cavendish, who worked with me on shaping the book you now have into your hands. Without his knowledge, experience, expertise and humour, this book would have been a very different one.

- To Marshall Cavendish, for having the faith in asking me to write a book and having the belief that Singaporeans would be receptive to such a book.

- To my parents for unconditionally loving and supporting me, for showing by example what it means to be good, what is love, courage and never giving up on life.

- To my friends Pearly Phua, Lim Seow Yuin, Wang Hongjun and Boey Yeong Kit, for knowing everything about me and still loving me, for always having my back and being real with me.

- To all my teachers for laying foundations on which I now stand, for being great at what you do, and for inspiring me to be the same.

- To all naysayers whom I have ever met who told me I cannot, could not, should not and must not, for helping me gain clarity more quickly about what I wanted to do and who I must become.

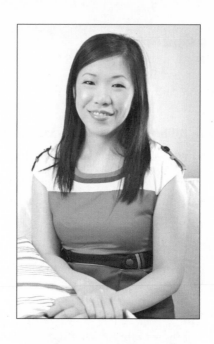

About the Author

Dr Martha Lee is Founder and Clinical Sexologist of Eros Coaching in Singapore. She provides sexuality and intimacy coaching for individuals and couples, conducts regular sexual education workshops and has spoken at public events in Asia and beyond. She is a certified sexuality educator with AASECT (American Association of Sexuality Educators, Counselors and Therapists), as well as a certified sexologist with ACS (American College of Sexologists). She holds a Doctorate in Human Sexuality from the Institute for Advanced Study of Human Sexuality as well as certificates in practical counselling, life coaching and sex therapy.

Often cited in the local media, Dr Lee is the appointed sex expert for *Men's Health Singapore* and *Men's Health Malaysia*. She has a column with PublicHouse.sg and blogs for *Good Vibrations Magazine*. She was recognised as one of "Top 50 Inspiring Women under 40" by *Her World* magazine in July 2010, and as one of "Top 100 Inspiring Women" by CozyCot in March 2011.

For more information, visit http://www.ErosCoaching.com.
Dr Martha Lee can be contacted at the following email:
drmarthalee@eroscoaching.com